Forget Burial

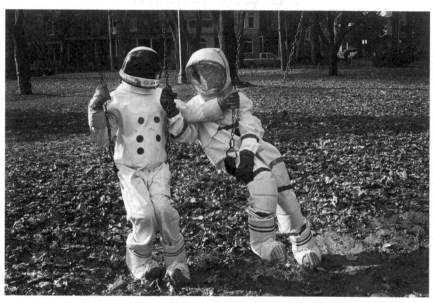

Frontispiece Jessica Whitbread (HIV activist) and Morgan M. Page (trans activist) having a date in spacesuits—also hazmat suits. Due to HIV stigma, Jessica feels she is constantly explaining to her dates that they don't need to wear spacesuits to have sex. From Jessica Whitbread and Morgan M. Page's photo series *Space Dates*. Courtesy of Jessica Whitbread and Morgan M. Page. Photo credit: Tania Anderson.

Forget Burial

HIV Kinship, Disability, and Queer/Trans Narratives of Care

MARTY FINK

RUTGERS UNIVERSITY PRESS
NEW BRUNSWICK, CAMDEN, AND NEWARK,
NEW JERSEY, AND LONDON

Library of Congress Cataloging-in-Publication Data

Names: Fink, Marty, author.
Title: Forget burial : HIV kinship, disability, and queer/trans narratives of care / Marty Fink.
Description: New Brunswick, New Jersey : Rutgers University Press, [2020] | Revision of author's thesis (doctoral)—City University of New York, 2010. | Includes bibliographical references and index.
Identifiers: LCCN 2020004899 | ISBN 9781978813779 (hardcover) | ISBN 9781978813762 (paperback) | ISBN 9781978813786 (epub) | ISBN 9781978813793 (mobi) | ISBN 9781978813809 (pdf)
Subjects: LCSH: HIV-positive persons—Care—United States—Historiography. | Caregivers—United States—Archives. | Caregivers—United States—Biography. | HIV-positive persons—Archives. | HIV-positive persons—Biography. | Sexual minorities with disabilities—United States—Historiography. | Sexual minority community—United States—Historiography. | Kinship care—United States—Historiography.
Classification: LCC RC606.6 .F56 2020 | DDC 362.19697/9200973—dc23
LC record available at https://lccn.loc.gov/2020004899

A British Cataloging-in-Publication record for this book is available from the British Library.

♾ The paper used in this publication meets the requirements of the American National Standard for Information Sciences—Permanence of Paper for Printed Library Materials, ANSI Z39.48-1992.

www.rutgersuniversitypress.org

Manufactured in the United States of America

For all the HIV heroes, mentors, and ghosts

Contents

Forget Burial

Introduction

TAKING CARE

In the summer of 1990, HIV activist and sex work organizer Iris De La Cruz performed a daring act at the New York University (NYU) Medical Center. With the support of fellow activists, she strategized to enter unnoticed into the hospital rooms of people living with HIV. Her campaign began in the middle of the night. When everyone was sleeping, and the hospital staff was otherwise engaged, De La Cruz proceeded toward the occupied beds. Undetectable until the following morning, the effects of her plan were set into motion. De La Cruz silently proceeded to decorate all the IV poles with pink ribbons and balloons, so that "everyone woke up to party IVs" (112). As De La Cruz reflects, "I had a good time getting this disease and I'm going to have a good time dealing with it." De La Cruz's narratives—which circulated in queer community newsletters, grassroots feminist publications, and activist videotapes—"reframe" (Hallas 3) HIV not as a "site of shame" (Erickson, "Revealing" 42) but as a site of community formation. This book begins with a hospital surprise party to bring HIV histories and contemporary disability movements together. I return to early HIV archives from the 1980s and 1990s to foreground stories of caregiving. These archives uncover how early HIV caregiving narratives continue to expand how we think about bodies in the present.

HAVING A GOOD TIME GETTING THIS DISEASE

I wrote this book to learn more about the work of De La Cruz and other HIV activists who died of AIDS in the 1980s and early 1990s. These HIV narratives transformed how I understand my own body, my experience of becoming disabled, and how I give and receive care. In sharing this project with my communities and with my students, I realized that many young people are deeply interested in these legacies but have little access to these early narratives about HIV. I began this research in 2006, when at age twenty-three I became keen to understand more about my own chosen families and our histories as queer and trans people. My intention was to create an opportunity for a generation that lost lovers, friends, and family to AIDS to pass down their experiences to those like myself who are continually looking to this older generation to make sense of our own bodies and our relationships to sexuality, to gender, and to HIV. This book's central argument is that literary and archival narratives of HIV caregiving offer a model of disability kinship that supports ongoing sexual and gender self-determination into the present. I wrote this book for my generational peers and for youth who do not yet have access to early HIV narratives. This work reflects my own desire to connect with the older generations who fought by learning about how I am personally impacted by their experiences of love and loss.

HIV and Disability

In this section, I consider how early HIV narratives shape cultural understandings of disability in the present. I return to caregiving narratives by activists including De La Cruz in order to reframe disability not as a problem with individuals' bodies but as a problem of institutions failing to care for the self-determination of disabled people. In countering narratives of pity and victimization, caregiving reframes HIV as inspiring how we might "love each other and support each other" (Shakur) in response to state refusal to care about HIV. As HIV activist and artist David Wojnarowicz famously declares, "I know I'm not going to die because I got fucked in the ass without a condom or because I swallowed a stranger's semen. If I die it is because a handful of people in power, in organized religions and political institutions, believe that I am expendable" (230). HIV narratives including Wojnarowicz's autobiography replace stigmatizing stories about disability with narratives of disability as the outcome of structural access barriers. As Alison Kafer observes of the process of describing disability, "Collective affinities in terms of disability could encompass everyone from people with learning disabilities to those with chronic illness, from people with mobility impairments to those with HIV/AIDS, from people with sensory impairments to those with mental illness. People within each of these categories can all be discussed in terms of disability politics, not because of any essential similarities among them, but because all have been labeled as disabled or sick and have faced discrimination as a result" (11). In widening the definition of disability to address discrimination, Robert McRuer also argues that disability studies should include HIV activism as a central component of its public histories. By claiming 1980s–'90s HIV activism as part of 1980s–'90s disability movements, McRuer advocates for "broadening, in public, our still-fluctuating sense of what disability history might be" ("Disability" 54). Drawing overt links between disability and HIV resists assimilationist and capitalist politics by leveraging "productively unruly bodies"

(McRuer, "Critical" Investments" 236) toward confronting ableist normalcy, increasing access to public space, and building antiracist coalitions (McRuer, "Critical Investments" 236, 230, 226; Linton 162–63; Sandahl 50; Stockdill 62; Farrow, "When My Brother Fell"). By regarding HIV as a disability, the caregiving activism to meet access needs, to counter stigma, and to connect individual body problems to larger struggles for antiracism, access to health care, and decolonization links ongoing histories of HIV activism to broader transnational movements (Bell et al. 439; Hobson, *Lavender* 3; Hobson, "Thinking" 205). Early HIV archives can be connected to ongoing queer and trans disability movements to support the self-determination of those who fail to conform to body norms.

These coalitions that link HIV and disability are, however, not without accompanying frictions. Alexander McClelland and Jessica Whitbread contextualize how some people living with HIV are reluctant to identify HIV activism with disability activism and its histories. McClelland and Whitbread identify the "past and existing tensions" (87) of framing HIV as disability. They illustrate that for people living with HIV, many of these conflicts "are unresolvable and, for some, highly personal" (87). They maintain, however, that understanding HIV as disability helps to address the criminalization of HIV nondisclosure in our contemporary moment (80). Citing disability activist and theorist AJ Withers, McClelland and Whitbread argue for the utility of reading HIV as disability in order to counter biomedical narratives and forms of state control that attempt to construct the "responsible" subject living with HIV as one who complies with able-bodied, "healthy" norms (92); McClelland and Whitbread analogously regard people living with HIV and other forms of disability as agents in resisting this process of state intervention toward self-defining "what it means to live with HIV in the contemporary context" (McClelland and Whitbread 85; Arsenault 2012; Chevalier and Bradley-Perrin). Considering HIV as disability also emphasizes the points of connection for all bodies marked as falling outside of medical norms. While some activists argue that disability can be understood as a positive and valuable form of diversity in the human condition, others have argued that disability is not always experienced positively because living with a disability can be the source of suffering, death, and pain (Wendell, "Unhealthy" 23; Mollow 76; Baril 60; Crow 61). Experiencing disability, further, does not always result in care. In fact, experiencing a lack of care when already vulnerable is what might cause our bodies to become disabling. Yet, disability creates opportunities for care and for feeling positive about body differences, even though—because of ableism and access barriers—it is not always experienced as such. HIV narratives can restore value and agency to bodies marginalized on account of being disabled. I therefore revisit early HIV caregiving archives alongside ongoing disability narratives that refuse to render certain bodies as expendable.

This book focuses on HIV in particular in order to better understand the sexual and gendered narratives attached to disability more generally. What I refer to as the "early" period of HIV begins in 1981 when HIV was first observed clinically in the United States, and ends in 1996 when the availability of antiretroviral drugs (to those with medical access and other forms of privilege) upset narratives of HIV as necessitating death; much work, however, has troubled this timeline of HIV history, as numerous activists and scholars have noted that just as the existence of HIV unquestionably predates 1981, so too are countless lives affected by HIV along lines of race and class in ways that have not improved since 1996 (Kerr, "AIDS 1969"; Robinson, "Homophobia" 9; Reid-Pharr ix; Gremk 105). I look to early responses to HIV rather than to broader instances of community-based caregiving; while I could also investigate queer and trans community responses to other crises in other historical periods, I am particularly interested in how early HIV narratives specifically offer models of anticonformist, gender fluid, anticapitalist, antiracist, and sex positive possibilities for reframing disability. The generational meanings connoted by the terms "HIV" and "AIDS" are also reflected at a linguistic level within my own writing. Unless I am explicitly discussing the syndrome "AIDS," I generally use the term "HIV" rather than "HIV/AIDS" to discuss the virus, its activisms, and its cultural meanings. While the term "HIV/AIDS" is the iteration of this acronym with which readers might be most familiar, I have decided to untether "HIV" from "AIDS" in my own usage to signify a shift across time, as "HIV" without "AIDS" marks a linguistic shift toward focusing not on the "pastness" of AIDS histories (Juhasz and Kerr) but rather on emphasizing HIV's ongoing meaning for people living with the virus. Through this linguistic choice, I also attempt to frame the process of living with HIV as ongoing, resisting a "false and dangerous dichotomy between past and present" (Aldarondo et al. 189). This contemporary use of the term "HIV" instead of "HIV/AIDS" is a linguistic decision that can be controversial. Some people prefer the term "AIDS" to refer to activist histories, and some prefer the term "HIV/AIDS," using the binary to separate HIV from AIDS without excluding the lived experience of either. Activists including Benjamin Ryan, however, prefer the use of the term "HIV" to counter institutional uses of the term "AIDS" in ways that erase the ongoing daily realities and activisms of people living with HIV today. The use of "HIV" over "HIV/AIDS" is thus intended as a linguistic move that roots these histories of AIDS as ongoing into HIV's present. In place of the term "people with AIDS" (PWAs), I use the term "people living with HIV" not to exclude people with AIDS or long term survivors from this category but because this term "HIV" feels useful as a linguistic refusal to locate these narratives as existing only with AIDS or only in the past.

CHOSEN FAMILIES AND HIV KINSHIPS

This section positions HIV in particular and disability more broadly as opportunity for queer and trans kinship. As someone who came of age with narratives of my own gender and sexuality as being inextricably linked to HIV stigma and sexual risk, I have always longed to transform these very narratives of pathologization into opportunities for finding family and exchanging care. Early HIV narratives offer my generation a way of understanding how our own queer-ness and trans-ness—and that of the chosen families we form to sustain us—are shaped by HIV and activist responses to it (Marcus 192; Sedgwick 184; Foucault 54; Delany, "Gamble" 140, 169; Elman 318; McCaskell 230; Sears 97; N. Nixon 128; Grover 23; Black and Whitbread 4; Joynt and Hoolbloom 26). I understand HIV "kinship" as different from simple "care" because while people can receive care in ways that are not necessarily connective, early HIV activism created what Mia Mingus terms "access intimacies." As Mingus outlines, access intimacies are a "tool for liberation" that "tap into the transformative powers of disabilities" by bringing people together precisely because of the connections that disability affords (Mingus; Erickson, "Revealing" 46; Rose 244). In forming these kinships in response to state violence, early HIV narratives offer this model of caregiving as forming these anticapitalist, antiableist kinships toward transforming access. In sharing this research with younger generations than mine, I also hope to model how HIV caregiving in particular has much to teach us about queer and trans survival. I apply HIV histories to contemporary narratives about gender and disability: rather than striving to cure disabilities and eliminate bodily differences, HIV narratives offer queer and trans models for taking care of each other when we experience institutional harm.

This book thus places early HIV archives in conversation with contemporary texts to present an ongoing model of queer and trans kinships that form in response to disability. "Queer" and "trans" are constantly evolving terms that when applied to the 1980s and 1990s may be anachronistic. Our present lens for understanding sexual and gender classifications differs from the ways in which these identities were understood historically. However, these umbrella terms are also useful for investigating how early HIV narratives influence contemporary understandings of these categories themselves. Juana Maria Rodriguez identifies not only that HIV is connected to intersecting oppressions on the basis of race, class, gender, and sexuality but that these dynamic categories of identity are shaped by the differences and affinities called into relief by HIV and its activisms (Rodriguez 47; Gould 215; Hobson, *Lavender* 193; Chen 196, 61; Stryker, *Transgender* 133; Gould 260; Johnson 148; Muñoz, *Disidentifications* 68, 151; Carroll 118; Joynt and Hoolbloom 90). Quo-Li Driskill further argues that while historians have positioned "queer" as emerging in the late 1980s and early 1990s out of political movements including HIV activism, two-spirit scholars have noted that "queer" has its formation not in the twentieth century but in the precolonial practices of indigenous communities prior to contact with white settlers (71).

TRANS LEGACIES AND HIV ARCHIVING

Forget Burial re-centers the work of trans women whose contributions to HIV histories have been frequently underrepresented both within mainstream retellings and within queer archiving practices. In the 1980s and 1990s, trans women supported other trans women living with HIV and responded to the needs of their communities, which were not addressed by "queer" HIV activists (M. Page, "Odofemi"; Mackay, "TRANSSEXUALS" 23). Morgan M. Page critiques canonized HIV activists including Vito Russo for trying to prevent Sylvia Rivera from speaking during an early 1970s Pride demonstration in New York City, excluding trans women of color from movements that trans women of color ignited via the Stonewall Riots. Rivera's work in the 1970s undertook a critical form of caregiving with the creation of Street Transvestite Action Revolutionaries (STAR) with Marsha P. Johnson as a form of care work to support and to house trans youth (Rivera 72). Che Gossett references the work of Tourmaline that re-centers these legacies of deliberately excluded Stonewall veterans—trans women of color—within HIV histories. Gossett reminds us that Johnson, leader of the gay liberation movement and the Stonewall riots, was "living with HIV and also cared for those close to her who were living with HIV, many of whom died during the onset of the AIDS epidemic" (Gossett and O'Malley 22). This early work of trans women is often excluded from HIV archives, an exclusion that continues to impact contemporary queer and trans community formations.

This project therefore looks not only for what is present in the HIV archive but also for what is missing. Archivists and scholars including Steven G. Fullwood, Kate Eichhorn, and Ann Cvetkovich identify the unpaid emotional labor of caring enough to collect, house, and look after archives across time and space (Cvetkovich 8; Eichhorn 14; Fullwood 48, 52; Sawdon-Smith, "Artists' Statement"; Carlomusto et al., *COMPULSIVE PRACTICE*). Jih-Fei Cheng also uncovers the labor of collective HIV activist video makers in caring for their footage to create cultures of memory, police accountability, and caregiving that support direct action (Bell et al. 86). The HIV archive thus also holds the potential to structure cultural production and labor collectively around forms of exchange that undercut capitalism (Eichhorn 10, 14–15; Cheairs et al. 6, 11; Hartman 228; Hobart and Kneese 8; E. Edelman 112; Hwang 570). While some HIV histories have been effectively preserved, others have become "degraded" (McKinney and Meyer).[1] I thus revisit

1. "Tape Condition: Degraded," Cait McKinney and Hazel Meyer's 2016 pornography exhibition at the ArQuives (a queer/trans national archive in Toronto's gay village), raises these questions of how histories of queer sex positivity (and porn) can be preserved through digitization from degraded VHS cassettes. McKinney and Meyer imagine these histories into existence while also lamenting the gap in findable materials other than those of commercial, gay, white productions. In failing to find the porn that they desire, McKinney and Meyer build, perform, draw, and collaborate with queer and trans artists to conjure porn that, in contributor Page's words, "dream of an archive in which bodies like mine and people who fuck like I do exist."

HIV archives not only to analyze what one might find there but also to inter-
rogate absence, taking care to question which caregiving testimonies have not
yet been sought out (Köppert and Sekuler; Youngblood; Fullwood 52; Namaste,
"AIDS" 139). McKinney traces the ongoing impact of revisiting untold historical narratives of HIV. In "Can a Computer Remember AIDS?" McKinney discusses the HIV archiving process, identifying how, "as archival logics order
cultural memory, they render certain 'AIDS of the past' intelligible, often at the
expense of others." Telling and retelling easily accessible stories can obscure the
violence of erasing histories that are harder to find (Patton, "Forward" x; Aldarondo et al. 194; Namaste, "AIDS" 141). In "AIDS 1969: HIV, History, and Race,"
Ted Kerr outlines how the HIV cases from 1981 that are often narrated as marking the beginning of HIV in North America obscure the legacies and access
needs of communities that were affected by HIV decades before this historical
moment. Kerr identifies that the media and medical professionals' inability to
notice or care about HIV until it began affecting white people creates a limited
narrative of HIV that continues into the present: "We keep repeating the history
we think we know to be true, the one that starts in 1981. But this is not the history
of HIV/AIDS; it is the history of our response to HIV/AIDS." Kerr reminds us
that telling narratives of these histories in the present "is powerful because it
shares stories about the AIDS crisis that inform the world we live in now." Thus
rather than re-creating what Chris Bell terms "White Disability Studies" (275)
by retelling the same—white-dominated, trans-exclusionary, already-told—
histories over again (Cheng, "AIDS" 77; Namaste, "AIDS" 131), this book follows
the advice of British Visual AIDS curator, historian, and photographer Ajamu,
who reframes HIV archiving as a dynamic process that "coincide[s] with other
moments across time, space, Diaspora" ("Gettin'"). As Ajamu asserts, "how we
think about archives is not what we go to but it's what we bring with us. How do
we bring ideas of pleasure, passions into archival work?" In attempting to answer
some of these questions, I return to HIV archives hoping these disability legacies
"can be lived and imagined a little differently" (Titchkosky 10) through a framework of mutual care. While care is not the only outcome or only possible reading of the archives I revisit, I center caregiving in order to preserve the work of
those who were lost, as well as the ongoing care that is taken in "remembering
and not remembering" (Varghese 2016), "to shovel dirt upon dirt upon dirt to bury
all the dead" (Robinson, "Archeology" 76), as survivors continue to mourn, to
memorialize, and to forget (Robinson, "Archeology" 75).

TAKING BACK CARE

Care is a central thread across this project that brings together early HIV activisms with contemporary disability kinships. In this section, I attempt to define
care with the same openness and flexibility with which care can be given.

Through early HIV narratives, I imagine an ongoing antiracist, antiassimilation-ist model of queer and trans care that disability movements can draw on to confront the access barriers created by capitalism. At its best, care can become a reciprocal process of mutual aid that forms queer and trans intimacies and familial connections as is evidenced by the activist responses to HIV (Bell et al. 439; Black and Whitbread 4). These HIV narratives, however, also uncover dis-appointments about inadequate care and the harm that occurs when care fails. HIV narratives thus further expose the ways in which capitalism and neoliber-alism, racism and colonialism, and anti-queer and anti-trans violence create bar-riers to giving and receiving mutual care (Bell et al. 455; Farber 181; Jolivette 238). A decolonial practice of caregiving, argues Juno Salazar Parreñas, also con-siders "how to relate to others beyond tired colonial tropes of violence and benevolence" (Parreñas 7); "decolonization is to be oriented toward process and experimentation and not toward a foregone conclusion, except for the need to care enough about others, including and in particular nonhuman others" (Parreñas 7). While care *giving* is essential for those whose access needs are not otherwise met by institutions including biological family and the medical system, this book thinks through the feminist possibility of care *taking*, of taking matters of body self-determination into "Our Own Hands."[2]

Forget Burial revisits these narratives of queer and trans intimacies that formed when care was denied by the state. The failure of the state in providing adequate care for people living with HIV reflects broader systems of gendered racism and colonialism perpetuated by capitalism (Singleton 51; Hobson, "Think-ing" 205). While grassroots queer and trans community care became necessary because of state neglect, the (albeit often inadequate) state systems that (can) exist to provide paid caregiving for disabled people eventually became available to people living with HIV. The shifts in care from grassroots supports to state sys-tems reflect the complexities and limits of providing care through capitalism (Hobson, "Thinking" 206). Emily Hobson, a historian of queer U.S. and radical movements, further links HIV activism and its histories to the ongoing "neo-liberal replacement of the state by non-governmental organizations (NGOs)" (Hobson, "Thinking" 206). Hobson's work challenges us to revisit HIV history not merely to romanticize the past but to connect HIV caregiving to addressing larger instances of racism, commodification, and global access barriers called into relief by paid caregiving, state disability services, and the nonprofit indus-trial complex ("Thinking" 206). As HIV caregiving theorists including Katie Hogan and Jeanine DeLombard point out, the majority of HIV caregiving labor is underpaid and unpaid and is provided domestically and/or through the state

2. *In Our Own Hands* is a collectively written feminist column about women and HIV from *Outweek* magazine (1989–1991) in which lesbian communities share information about resource access. I unburied these periodicals at the Lesbian Herstory Archives in 2008, and the collection has since been digitized and is now available online.

by queer and BIPOC (black, indigenous, people of color) women (Hogan 4; DeLombard 351). Moreover, daily experiences of racism, job precarity, and low wages are characteristic of state-funded paid labor within domestic care, nursing, and long-term care institutions (Ryosho 60; Bauer and Cranford 66; Hobart and Kneese 8). An analysis of early HIV caregiving models created in opposition to capitalism thus can offer broader ongoing interventions in disability caregiving toward "addressing racism . . . translating personal analysis into collective political action and thus simultaneously transforming both individuals and social institutions" (Ryosho 68). Rather than simply advocating for caregiving without the state or for adopting a caregiving model that is state-run, this book instead understands caregiving as a framework through which to critique capitalism itself for failing to provide care in a nonexploitative way. As disability justice writer and activist Leah Lakshmi Piepzna-Samarasinha argues in *Care Work: Dreaming Disability Justice*, DIY (do-it-yourself) models of care from the everyday lives of queer and trans people of color offer alternatives to racist and gendered state systems by "break[ing] from the model of paid attendant care as the only way to access disability support" (41). Lakshmi Piepzna-Samarasinha challenges neoliberal models of caregiving toward the anarchist crip goal of radically "rewriting of what care means, of what disability means" (46) by mapping out queer and trans of color community care webs "controlled by the needs and desires of the disabled people running them" (41). In placing early HIV caregiving narratives in conversation with these contemporary movements, *Forget Burial* revisits ongoing legacies of HIV activism not simply to create a new model of care but to disrupt the labor norms of capitalism.

Returning to early HIV narratives of caregiving thus offers an ongoing critique of capitalism for undervaluing care work. In *The Erotic Life of Racism*, Sharon Holland draws on queer and critical race theory to "take care of the feeling" (6) that "escapes or releases" (6) as bodies "collide in pleasure and in pain" (6); Holland understands desire and intimacy as informing daily acts of racism, and therefore urges readers to care about the feelings that this process creates (11). In reading early HIV narratives as offering anticapitalist, antiracist caregiving models that value the access needs, desires, and labor practices of communities of color (Lakshmi Piepzna-Samarasinha 46), the queer and trans exchanges of pleasure and pain in these narratives contest the state forms of care and the kinds of racism that state systems—and state caregiving systems in particular—continue to perpetuate. Drawing on Loree Erickson's queer and trans caregiving collectives, Lakshmi Piepzna-Samarasinha asks, "What does it mean to shift our ideas of access and care . . . from an individual chore, an unfortunate cost of having an unfortunate body to a collective responsibility that's maybe even deeply joyful?" (33). *Forget Burial* revisits these joys not merely to wax nostalgic about early HIV narratives but to grapple with the contradictions and complexities of community caregiving to imagine these anticapitalist possibilities into the future.

A return to early HIV archives also reframes caregiving as a form of activism. Because caregiving labor is often gendered and unpaid, it can become dismissed as being less revolutionary than now-iconic forms of HIV street protest. This book analyzes novels and other caregiving narratives to re-center many different kinds of care as frontline work. These narratives demonstrate how forming chosen families—as well as transforming how we understand and treat our biological families—has always been a vital response to the failure of capitalist systems in providing adequate support. HIV archives also attest to the ongoing racism and colonialism of the state, and to community responses to institutional access barriers to care. The antiblack racism enacted through medical access barriers is addressed in a 1986 archival issue of *Black/Out*, a black gay newsletter published in Philadelphia. In this newsletter, black gay literary anthologizer and editor Joseph Beam, who was living with HIV, writes, "The State (a euphemism for white people) has never been concerned with the welfare of Black people. . . . It is not a matter of whether their racism is intentional or unintentional. We die 'by accident' daily and the State is a witness who documents that demise." Beam quotes the poetry of Essex Hemphill to encourage black communities to take health issues into their own hands: "Hemphill writes in 'For My Own Protection': We should be able to save each other / I don't want to wait for the Heritage Foundation to release a study saying / Black people are almost extinct." The 1986 publication *Bebashi: Blacks Educating Blacks about Sexual Health Issues*, also published prior to the formation of late-1980s movements like ACT UP, already identifies how "AIDS is a disease, not a lifestyle. And the methods through which it spreads are no longer a mystery or hard to explain. But the socio-political reality is that those who have traditionally had greater access to health care and educational opportunities are those who today are learning how to protect themselves against this disease. And those who are traditionally forgotten are again being forgotten—with tragic, almost genocidal consequences" ("AIDS and Minorities" 2).

Early HIV-chosen families thus formed in response to the failures of biological families and the state (Knauer 162; N. Nixon 128; Greyson 1987; Gillett 9–10; Wolfe 227; Foege 616; Bryan 69; Kramer 20; Denneny 42). This grassroots response to state medical negligence is one in which black, indigenous, and other underserved communities have always created in order to meet their own medical needs (L. Nixon 2017; S. Smith 169; Konsmo 2013; Wilson 81; Yee 22; Oliver et al. 909; Hewitt 9; Woubshet 43; Dryden). When connected to these long histories of community-centered care provision—and to emerging disability movements—HIV caregiving narratives become part of an ongoing disruption to neoliberal systems that regard each of us as responsible for our own health (Clare, *Brilliant* 9; Derkatch, "Self-Generating" 134; Derkatch, "'Wellness'" 6; Derkatch, *Bounding* 185; Geary 4; Hobart and Kneese 3). Using his own HIV test as a visual example of the medicalization of the individual gay male body, Samuel Delany expresses frustration with this medical rhetoric of testing through which "health itself is totally and forever denied but rather deferred, test after test after test, until, presumably, death" ("Gamble" 140). Delany addresses the cultural imperative toward health by weaving risk into his life's narrative and by managing it as a calculated component of his relationship to cruising. Delany writes, "I enjoy a certain kind of pleasure. I gamble on getting it" ("Gamble" 169). In opposition to such individualist understandings of "health," HIV narratives of caregiving re-center the gendered labor and the queer and trans communities formed while fighting for disability access.

Revisiting HIV archives thus also offers an ongoing narrative of queer and trans responses to state medical violence into the present. These narratives reframe disabled bodies as inspiring the formation of kinships rather than as "sites of shame" (Erickson, "Revealing" 42). De La Cruz's autobiographical accounts of leading some of the first-ever support groups for women living with HIV, of decorating hospital rooms with birthday paraphernalia, and of hosting (and writing about) HIV Passover Seders exemplify this narrative reframing: De La Cruz depicts her own experience in the hospital not as a source of shame but as one of gay-famous celebrity sightings and mutual support. In the camp tradition of celebrity gossip, she reports, "Well, low and behold! The guys hanging out read like a Who's Who of the HIV community. Sitting in the middle of all the madness, holding court, was my very own *Newsline* editor, Phil. And he was surrounded by some very impressive people, like the activists Vito Russo and Damien Martin and some other guys that aren't gonna talk to me 'cause I didn't mention them here" ("Invasion" 111). Inverting the stigma of recognition, De La Cruz identifies the opportunities for queer friendship and sexual affirmation that can be found in the hospital ward. Contesting cultural representations of disability as a desexualized site of shame, De La Cruz creates community-driven forums to express desire for bodies living with HIV: "I'm going to kick off a new idea in the *Newsline*; it's going to be called the hot PWA of the month. So, if you have any photos of yourself or your buddies to send them in with a paragraph or two about yourself, we'll run it." Inverting mainstream media narratives of stigma and contagion, De La Cruz cautions to "please make sure you have at least minimal clothing on, (although I'd be more than happy to accept nudes for my own personal use) because the *Newsline* doesn't need an obscenity suit." In building community via the "hot PWA," De La Cruz's work speaks back to narratives that position disability as antithetical to sexual desire. As Erickson argues, disability holds the potential to bring queer crip bodies together "to create and find places where we are appreciated and celebrated for the very differences that are often used to justify our oppression" (42). Drawing on Erickson's work, I lean into the possibilities for caregiving to be sexy and connective rather than necessarily isolating, underappreciated, or an inevitable source of burnout. De La Cruz's claiming of the NYU Medical Center as a sexualized, queer social scene in the early 1990s speaks to the work of contemporary disability activists like Erickson and Withers who sexualize the "pleasure and shame" (Rees 112) of medical waiting rooms as cruising zones and make porn about wheelchairs in order to—like the HIV activists who preceded them—locate their queer crip bodies as prompting collective resistance.

JUST DROP MY BODY ON THE STEPS OF THE F.D.A.

In this next section, I consider my own relationship to early HIV kinships, in spite of the fact that I was too young in the 1980s and early 1990s to become part of this movement. Upon first entering the HIV archives to begin this project over a decade ago, I was not initially searching for stories about doing the dishes, listening, and food preparation. When I became an HIV activist in my twenties in the first decade of the 2000s, I was not expecting that my primary role in HIV community would be in doing the dishes, listening, and food preparation. What I was searching for in my HIV work—both as activist and as academic—was for stories of how the system fails to support queer and trans people. In learning how many of these stories are really about care, it became apparent that caregiving is also the organizing principle of my own work. This research does not merely point to the beauty and power of care but also makes unavoidable the failures and disappointments of becoming vulnerable with and to others. HIV archives capture moments when care becomes transformative against stigma and isolation but also when it does not. Caregiving narratives actually foreground the limitations and pain of bodies, of mourning, of burnout, of selling out, and of stories that remain forgotten, buried, and unresolved.

I revisit these HIV narratives not just in spite of the fact that I was not involved but precisely in response to this knowledge gap in my own generational experience: how am I impacted by this legacy of community care that I am not able to personally know? In connecting early HIV caregiving narratives to gender and sexuality in the present, I revisit a portrait of Wojnarowicz that continues to circulate across print and digital platforms.[3] Photographed by Bill Dobbs at an ACT UP protest of the Food and Drug Administration (FDA) in 1988, Wojnarowicz sports a denim jacket with a pink triangle on the back. Printed in DIY large white block letters on the back of the jacket, the bold script scrawled loudly

3. For instance, on Tumblr this image's circulation between April and July 2014 alone produced upwards of 60,691 likes and reposts. The 2012 re-creation of this denim jacket by youth including photographer and textile crip artist Katie Jung attests to its ongoing resonance. This photograph was also circulated in *Corpus*, an HIV publication by AIDS Project Los Angeles in 2006 (Ayala 80). In conversation with Jean Carlomusto in *Corpus*, photographer Every Ocean Hughes also discusses her tribute to Wojnarowicz's body through her own self-portraits, as she expresses her desire: "To work with David, stitch myself into bed with him, turn myself into a fag. Yes, turn myself into a fag, allow my desire to move my body, change my body, to make something that gets me closer" (Carlomusto and Hughes 78).

across Wojnarowicz's body relays the message "If I die of AIDS—forget burial—just drop my body on the steps of the F.D.A." The imperative here is not to forget "my" individual burial but rather to embody a collective refusal by people living with HIV to "disappear quietly" (Wojnarowicz 230). Wojnarowicz showcases the power of his own sick body and even his corpse in forcing a homophobic system to care about HIV (Anonymous Queers 1992; Feinberg 264). I play—in this book's title and in its content—with the narrative meanings of "burial" to address the ongoing state violence that marks certain bodies as undeserving of access to care (Nguyen 4; J. H. Jones 109; Herndl 555; Cohen 36; S. L. Smith 5, 113; Washington 400; Crimp 133; Sharpe 50; Dryden). Unburying these narratives of loss directs accountability toward institutions that devalue the survival of bodies that do not conform. Archives of caregiving also "forget burial" by preserving across generations the narratives of those who have died (Gill-Peterson, "Haunting" 280; Castiglia and Reed 9; Arriola; Hilderbrand 307; Woubshet x, 24).

Although it remains tempting to affirm the pervasive narrative that older queers are responsible for dispensing these histories to a disappointingly apathetic younger audience (Finkelstein, "Silence = "), this simplified assumption of disconnect between generations is often inaccurate; such narratives of disconnect obscure how HIV caregiving and its historical preservation are already happening—and have always been happening—across generational lines (Barnhardt 13). Juhasz and Kerr identify the utility of "rubbing the past up against the present" to consider what out-of-circulation media mean to young viewers in current contexts. Juhasz calls this process "queer archive activism" ("Video Remains" 320), which refers to using video edits and one's own presence within the footage to "remember, feel anew, analyze, and educate, ungluing the past from its melancholic grip, and instead living it as a gift with others in the here and now" ("Video Remains" 326). These material archives also connect HIV activisms of the 1980s and 1990s with digital disability movements of the present. I therefore "forget burial" and unbury archives to ask how HIV histories offer disability kinship models that continue to support queer and trans body self-determination.

Bringing these HIV histories into the present necessarily emphasizes generational differences in lived experience, as well as barriers to witnessing trauma across generations. Visual AIDS curator and artist Nathan Lee and artist and writer Carlos Motta create dialogue to address these intergenerational challenges of attempting to access HIV histories as younger queer men. Lee and Motta discuss pre-exposure prophylaxis (PrEP) in the context of their own relationship to HIV. Writing to Motta, Lee recognizes, "I will never know what it means to live through the AIDS crisis. I will never watch all my friends get sick and die. The enormity of that experience is a kind of black box I cannot access. And that is something I've realized that I increasingly need to respect and account for in all my words and thoughts."

When I began my research for this book in the mid-2000s as a graduate student, my objective was to learn how to talk about HIV activist legacies in a way that could bring that experience of death and loss into a contemporary context. I thought that by studying hard and performing well, I could transmit the traumatic experiences of queer activists preceding me to my own generation, and that would make for an exciting research project. At the end of my oral exams that would qualify me to begin work on my dissertation, I awaited the remarks of a panel of legendary HIV activists (now also distinguished English professors), who all frowned at me from across the examination table. In a display of tough love, which I now understand as an act (very New York City) of care, my mentors clarified my central problem: *"Marty, it is clear from this exam how much you love literature and how much you love to read, but you know absolutely nothing about what it was like to live through those years of the AIDS crisis."* I learned in this moment that my project could never be about understanding HIV across generations. I realize now that I will never be able to comprehend what it means to live through (or die in) this period. I also learned from writing this book that my retelling of these archival stories will always be inaccurate precisely because I was not there. My decision, however, to nevertheless investigate this archive comes out of a persistent desire from my own generational experience of trying to make sense of what HIV is and how HIV activists, many of whom have died and I will never get to meet, change the way I continue to understand myself. The act of revisiting HIV archives of the 1980s and 1990s is, as Eichhorn acknowledges, "not . . . to recover the past but rather a way to engage with some of the legacies, epistemes, and traumas pressing down on the present" (5). As Christina Sharpe reflects: "I am interested in how we imagine ways of knowing that past, in excess of the fictions of the archive, but not only that. I am interested, too, in the ways we recognize the many manifestations of that fiction and that excess, that past not yet past, in the present" (14). In attempting to understand the present through this revisiting, I hope—as Lee and Motta advise—to continue to "try to grasp where the contours of my experience are structured by the *limitations* of my experience." As Eichhorn reminds us, "a turn toward the archive is not a turn toward the past but rather an essential way of understanding and imagining other ways to live in the present" (9). Similarly, Cvetkovich outlines, the project of uncovering HIV activist histories is as much one of building an archive as it is of examining one (8; Snorton 178). In unburying HIV archives, I reframe my own generational understanding of queer and trans kinship, of caregiving, and of disability in relation to this legacy of loss.

When I started this project, my first archival visit was to the HIV collections at the New York Public Library (NYPL). In her investigation of the NYPL's HIV archives, Cvetkovich captures the disconnect between the activist aesthetic of these cultural artifacts and the sterile finery of the NYPL's reading room wherein much of this archive is housed. The NYPL hosts one of the largest HIV archives, containing everything from collective meeting minutes documenting the grass-roots organizing of the Women's AIDS Resource Network (WARN) to activist David Feinberg's personal cookbook (and pornography) collections. The materials found in the HIV collections expand conceptions of what might constitute HIV "literature" and what might compose a disability "archive." Cvetkovich maps the various initial locations of the HIV archive prior to its ultimate arrival at the NYPL, where it remains to ensure its continued preservation. She then recounts her experience of accessing the archive: "The classical architectures and huge reading room are imposing, displaying on a massive scale the idea of tradition, which is being invented as well as preserved by the archive. Entry to the manuscript collection is available by special application only to those who have specific research projects; the research room, which is located off the main reading room, feels like a sequestered space for devoted, and slightly antiquated, scholars" (247). I noted this disconnect most heavily when—upon sitting at this marbled, ivoried, grandiose table of biblical scholars—I opened a box of Feinberg's porn. The contradiction between the unabashed sexual cultures of HIV activism and the sterilized material history inhabited by the dislocated researcher points to the possibilities for taking these collections out of their boxes and challenging contemporary disability narratives through their recirculation. This archive contains materials including the decoupaged index cards of Feinberg's favorite gay personal ads, as well as the unpublished "AIDS Journals, 1989–1992," of New York City–based artist, writer, and sculptor Stuart Edelson. Edelson's words directed me from the outset of my project to consider the experience of living with HIV in relation to disability. In his diary, Edelson discusses a dilemma he faces when he begins to feel too sick to work (Dyck 122; Withers, *Disability* 11). He writes, "I have a pretty good idea that the amount of money I would have to live on if I went on permanent disability, would be totally inadequate to cover my needs. I would be acquiring a new and worse disease called POVERTY! So I've decided to put that inevitability off for as long as I can. Let me embarrass or disgust them all into knowing how mean our system is." When I first read these words in Edelson's unpublished diaries, I felt moved to reprint them. To resist investigating this period as a static thing, I turn to HIV archives as inspiring an active process of curation. As *Corpus* editor Pato Hebert reminds us through his editorial work of curating queer, antiracist art and literature in support of sex education and body self-determination, "AIDS is a disaster. It is also an opportunity" (x). Rather than reading narratives of early HIV activism as already fixed in the past, this book recirculates these archives as ongoing opportunity to offer a narrative model of community caregiving toward addressing the persistent meanness of "our system."

SYSTEM MEANNESS, PRISON ABOLITION, AND COVID-19

As I complete this book during the initial months of the COVID-19 pandemic, I join my communities in drawing on the legacy of HIV activism to intervene, in Edelson's words, in "how mean our system really is." My hope is that *Forget Burial* can be useful in understanding COVID-19 as a disaster that is "also an opportunity" (Hebert x) to end capitalism, abolish prisons, and eliminate the police. In response to the colonial and racist increase in policing and surveillance with COVID-19, I also witness the widespread discussion of caregiving as it relates to access to safe housing, income support, decarceration, sex work decriminalization, overdose prevention, gender self-determination, and improved medical care, as well as to body self-determination, pleasure, sex, and risk (Mikiki, "We Can't Police"; Kerr, "How to Live"; McClelland, *We Can't Police*, "We Can't Police"; Dodd, *We Can't Police*; E. Jones; Davis; Wesley; Mutual Aid Disaster Relief; Juhasz "Introduction"; Ware; Walia; Hastings; Dryden; Kinsman; Jackson et al., Maynard and Ritchie). In *We Can't Police Our Way Out of the Pandemic*, Toronto-based activist and artist Mikiki Mikiki connects the current criminalization of queer sex and substance use during COVID-19 to the criminalization of HIV (Mikiki's HIV art and activism is also further discussed in chapter 1). Mikiki observes that we "have a long history as queer people of using whatever tools are available to . . . mitigate our internalized homophobia, the sex negativity that's forced on us, and also, our own trauma histories and I would also include within that the being raised as straight people and then failing as straight people, and doing that for a lot of us within the context of the other pandemic [laughs] of the HIV epidemic." Mikiki calls for the widespread challenging of media and cultural narratives that vilify queer men for seeking pleasure, for using substances, and for having sex during the time of COVID-19. Mikiki identifies how such narratives are being used to increase the policing, surveillance, and criminalization of those already targeted by colonial and racist state systems and by HIV criminalization laws; Mikiki also connects COVID-19 state violence to the Canadian government's current military occupation of the unceded Wet'suwet'en territory, an occupation set in place to build pipelines, destroy the environment, and deny indigenous sovereignty. These ongoing histories of colonialism and racism create cultural narratives about whose rights for self-determination are legitimate and whose should be contained. Mikiki connects COVID-19 narratives to the antiqueer and antitrans narratives underpinning the criminalization of HIV: "the seeking of pleasure and intimacy and connection which queer men are known for and will continue to be known for . . . is [seen as] inherently irresponsible at best and malicious at worst . . . seen as suicidal all the way to murderous." I therefore draw on Mikiki's analysis to link COVID-19 caregiving to the archives of HIV caregiving unburied in this book.

Early HIV narratives offer models of collective organizing that continue to shape queer and trans body self-determination in the present.

The caregiving kinships of early HIV activism offer narratives of queer and trans people forming family to support collective intimacies and insurgencies not in spite of, but because of disability. In coming together to meet their access needs, early HIV caregivers demanded medical justice on a systemic level. The archives revisited in *Forget Burial* demonstrate how medical access requires confronting and transforming state systems rather than leveraging individual blame or fear in response to disability. The early caregiving activist responses to HIV, including the invention of safer sex, reflect a history of queers working together at a grassroots level to research, collect, debate, and share sexual health information despite the blocking of these prevention initiatives by the state (Schulman, *My American History* 113; Patton, "Resistance and the Erotic" 70; Carlomusto, *Sex*; Berkowitz 2; DiAna, "DiAna's"; Patton, *Globalizing* 66; Gould 77; Brier 1; Pearl, *AIDS Literature* 64; Gould 66; Race 7). Drawing on HIV legacies in response to COVID-19, Mikiki asks queer community members today to again think through the question of "how do we look out for each other?" Mikiki argues that public health campaigns demanding that people abstain from sex and from substance use during COVID-19 is an untenable mode of public health intervention that fails to account for the ways in which the risk of viral transmission occurs not because of careless individual transgressions but because of the uneven distribution of access to housing, income, health care, safety, support, intimacy, community, and pleasure so that people can effectively "stay home" (Mikiki, *We Can't Police*; E. Jones; Dryden; Jackson et al; Maynard and Ritchie; Kinsman; Davis; Walia; Dodd, *We Can't Police*; McClelland, "We Can't Police"; Hastings): "people have needs and they're going to meet them because people have been finding ways to meet our needs that exist outside of state services, outside of capitalism . . . for numbers of years. The issue, I think, is about how to we hold these two ideas that can seem contraindicated or too disparate but it's this idea of—how do we support personal bodily autonomy and   how do we also hold ourselves and each other accountable to a collective idea of care and prevention." Early HIV narratives demonstrate the theory and the practice of this collective model of caregiving, where mutually exchanging care creates disability kinships that meet individual needs toward countering the systems that unequally distribute medical access.

Forget Burial's narratives of early HIV kinship further illustrate how the act of supporting queer and trans body self-determination shifts the onus away from the individual and onto the state. In our present moment of COVID-19, activists and scholars on social media are identifying the dangers of neoliberal models of caregiving that fail to transform the conditions that necessitate community care in response to a lack of accessible state care. As Shana Almeida identifies in a

Facebook post: "kindness as a political act is understanding and then actively dismantling the principles of capitalism which *require* poverty, to thrive. Or, at the very least, advocating for housing for all and that basic needs are met for everyone. The problem is, we want to have the power to say when and to whom we offer kindness. Our biggest problem is that, especially in the current political moment, we want our acts of kindness to cost us very little and also to be given in the most dire of circumstances. And then we want to be celebrated for those acts." Almeida's post implores readers to:

Make.

Your.

Kindness.

Political.

This caution that neoliberal forms of caregiving will sustain rather than transform the status quo, helps me articulate more clearly my own definition of caregiving in this book. As Almeida advocates in response to COVID-19, *Forget Burial* offers models of kinship and of mutual aid that although enacted by individuals, nevertheless collectively responds to disability by confronting the negligence of the state. As academic and community organizer Nisha Eswaran argues in an Instagram post, the current trend of academics to write about care in response to COVID-19 reinforces the very systems that disability holds the potential to challenge, "it's not surprising but I'm so . . . grumpy about the academic response to the crisis of the moment. Why are people returning to 'an ethics of care' instead of, I don't know, socialism which also includes an analysis of all the social reproduction work that low-wage and BIPOC women do so that academics can sit at home and write our . . . research projects that no one cares about? Redistribute your money and go wash dishes at the food bank . . . ! Don't @ me in defence of this because I'm mad." These critiques of neoliberal caregiving models and of the academic theorizing of care identify the importance of understanding medical violence as a problem that necessitates the transformation of social systems rather than merely modifying the behavior of individuals to compensate for the failure of the state.

This narrative practice of blaming individuals for the spread of disease is not new to COVID-19 but reflects a long, ongoing history of racist and colonial narratives of contagion (E. Jones; Dryden; Wesley; Kinsman; Walia; Davis). Holding individuals responsible for public health is a fallacy that HIV scholars have cautioned is unrealistic, untenable, and relies on an impossible logic system; as Julia Epstein argues, "this individualist explanation proposed that disease could be caused and/or exacerbated by deviant behavior, and such behavior could also result from the disease process—a lose-lose proposition, because deviance would make you sick but at the same time meant that you were already sick . . . leaving a chicken and egg problem with conflicted social implications" (J. Epstein, *Altered* 171; Dean 61; Brandt 161; Hoppe 44; Jordan-Zachery 121). This narrative misapplication of blame to the individual in COVID-19 is used to criminalize black, indigenous, and racialized people for not "adhering to physical distancing" (Dryden), meanwhile, this safety requirement for keeping six feet of physical distance—as black queer activist and scholar OmiSoore Dryden was informed by a police officer while he put his body aggressively close to hers on the street—"does not apply to police" (Dryden). The police brutality that directly increases COVID-19 transmission risk for those most vulnerable to policing, relies on these culturally entrenched disability narratives that blame individuals and not state systems for the spread of a virus (Mikiki, *We Can't Police*; Hastings; Maynard and Ritchie; Straube; Kinsman; Dryden; Walia; Wesley; Davis; E. Jones; McClelland, *We Can't Police*, "We Can't Police'"; Jackson et al; Dodd, *We Can't Police*; Ware). As poet, academic, and activist El Jones argues, the narrative that criminalizes people who risk transmitting COVID-19 for failing to physically distance not only targets those who lack the resources needed to safely "stay home" but this narrative of individual blame frames police and prisons as a solution to violence, in spite of the fact that policing and prisons increase rather than decrease harm (E. Jones; sachse 203; Spade 156; Ritchie, *Arrested* 4; Ben-Moshe et al. 14). As Jones explains, the failure of state justice systems for punishing individuals without addressing any of the social factors that cause individual acts of violence becomes undeniably apparent in COVID-19, "we'll have a reading of violence that says this person is committing violence, but then we don't read of course the police as violent, we don't read this bailout to corporations while people lose their businesses as an act as violence, we don't read keeping people in prison while COVID is spreading as violence, so we have this incredibly narrow view of violence that reads it as entirely committed by individuals and ignores all the forms of state, patriarchal, racist, colonial violence that influences every day."

Like HIV caregiving activism, Jones's analysis demonstrates how caregiving in response to COVID-19 can also reframe disability to newly think through the complex "grey areas" (Jones) of prison abolition. Like HIV, COVID-19 presents an opportunity to build tangible alternatives to police and to prison that also hold individuals accountable to each other as a form of caregiving (E. Jones; Ware; Mikiki, *We Can't Police*). As Jones identifies:

> The challenge of abolition is exactly this question . . . how can we be honest about the times when we feel vindictive, the times when we want punishment, the times when we've maybe had to call authorities, all of those things are really important in discussion . . . we cannot continue to use those things as stumbling blocks to doing the hard work to think past it . . . we have to be really willing to do that hard and complex work, to make those mistakes, and we also have to I think, finally, engage with people that have committed harm. People in prisons that are there for things like multiple murders and shootings have a lot of insight and understanding in how transformation works and

how accountability works and what remorse looks like . . . they have very clear ideas and have done a lot of work and they're some of our best sources in talking about what happened, why did this happen, and how do we change that? . . . and this is what happens when we create this idea of violence, is then those people get excluded from the very conversations that we need to be able to have.

In bridging COVID-19 organizing with prison abolition movements, Black Lives Matter Toronto artist, activist, and scholar Syrus Marcus Ware identifies: "one of the things Giselle Dias talks about a lot is this idea that abolition is rooted in indigenous resurgence, and is rooted in anticolonial work, and so that abolition is not just closing carceral spaces—including psychiatric detention and immigration detention—abolition is overthrowing capitalism on Turtle Island, and so this is where our work is beginning in earnest." *Forget Burial* returns to early HIV archives toward this abolitionist, anticapitalist objective of reframing disability as a site of power to transform the present. Unburying HIV narratives of queer and trans caregiving in this moment of COVID-19 reframes disability not as an individual body problem but as opportunity to hold each other, as Mikiki reminds us from behind a computer screen, pausing between sentences with laughter, "intimacy and pleasure are basic features of the human experience. I hope that's not news for anybody. And I think that we are going to find ways of connecting."

Having a Good Time Dealing with It

My methodology undertakes the literary analysis of novels alongside a multitude of other materials including theory, autobiographies, short stories, poetry, and nonfiction writing, as well as archives, oral histories, zines, visual art, video, porn, and digital media. Across the chapters of this book, I close read novels alongside this constellation of media to reimagine ongoing queer and trans responses to state violence and to the daily pain, grief, and care of navigating disability and death. Although current queer and trans theoretical frameworks for analyzing genders and sexualities did not yet exist in the 1980s and 1990s, their application to these archives inform my observations of how early HIV narratives influence ongoing narrative practices of resistance to ableist, hetero, white supremacist, colonial, and cisgender norms. While some of the contemporary texts I analyze address HIV directly, I argue how even those works that do not engage with HIV overtly can be placed in conversation with caregiving archives to challenge body norms.

In chapter 1, I ask what it would mean to read Octavia Butler's 2005 vampire novel *Fledgling* as a caregiving novel about HIV. In reimagining these queer, polyamorous, undead communities alongside archives of HIV, this chapter provides a framework for reading disability as a powerful site of kinship. Communities of care, Butler's novel reveals, are not utopias but contain the same gendered and racist violence reinforced by caregiving narratives themselves. These forms of harm, a caregiving reading of the novel uncovers, can be addressed through Afrofuturist reimaginings of justice. Through my literary analysis of *Fledgling*, this chapter also connects contemporary HIV activism to archives documenting the invention of safer sex. This chapter understands community accountability and obtaining consent as forms of caregiving that support autonomy from the state. Butler's work thus offers disability kinship models toward decriminalization and prison abolition.

Responding to the communal possibilities offered by Butler's vampires, chapter 2 revisits archival videos, poetry, newsletters, zines, and posters as narrative records of caregiving activism. This chapter recalls trans women's activist histories that have been excluded from HIV archival collections. Through narrative analysis, I revisit a variety of trans women's archives to observe the formation of queer community partnerships and fractures via HIV caregiving. This chapter considers the function of HIV activism in rebuilding broken coalitions between trans and gay communities, and in supporting trans-chosen family formation through the destigmatization of disability. In chapter 3, I move from chosen communities to the biological family as a critical site of care. I place a literary analysis of Sarah Schulman's HIV fiction in conversation with the contemporary short fiction of Casey Plett. These texts together with archival and contemporary writing by activists including De La Cruz, Bryn Kelly, and Sur Rodney (Sur) offer a host of representational possibilities for narrating disability kinships formed in response to family trauma. I read fiction alongside autobiographical writing to consider how the family can become a site of harm but can also sustain reciprocal care.

Chapter 4 then takes up an examination of Rebecca Brown's narrative strategies for representing the chosen families and queer intimacies that can emerge from caregiving. A lesbian writer whose 1994 publication *The Gifts of the Body* brought her from independent publishing venues into mainstream media outlets, Brown omits the biographical details of her unnamed narrator in this literary account of HIV care. Reading *The Gifts of the Body* alongside Brown's earlier HIV short story "A Good Man" (2003) raises questions of narrative withholding and of why Brown erases herself from her own autobiographically based text. Through this process of emotional distancing, the narrator actually demonstrates the interconnectivity between bodies that caregiving can create, building queer chosen families in response to HIV. Chapter 5 traces this phenomenon again in Jamaica Kincaid's *My Brother*, which likewise represents care through the perspective of a conspicuously misleading auto/biographer (the slash here conveys how writing another's story is ultimately a process of reflecting about oneself, and how one's own self-narrative is always constructed in relation to others). This chapter revisits Kincaid's deceptively straightforward (and deceptively straight) diasporic text, reconsidering the role (and the reliability) of the narrator in the act of giving care. I read this gap between this untrustworthy narrator persona and the author herself as exposing the barriers to care created by ongoing histories of slavery, colonialization, and forced migration. In reading Kincaid's work alongside the prison activism of AIDS Counseling and Education (ACE), HIV caregiving narratives again offer a framework for imagining prison abolition via disability kinships. In reading Kincaid's representations of queer family formations in conversation with early HIV documentaries of prison activism, this chapter uncovers the limits and failures—as well as the narrative openness and transformative potential—of care.

The chapters of this book thus begin with an abolitionist reading of Butler's speculative fiction about the creation of chosen families in response to disability, and end with ACE's real-life formation of HIV community in prison. The sequencing of the chapters presents a progression that considers the various successes and the disappointments of queer and trans caregiving as providing different kinds of intimacies in supporting decriminalization, prison abolition, and defunding the police. In observing representations of HIV family formations, their aspirations toward mutual care, and their inevitable limitations, I argue that bringing early HIV narratives into present continues to shape our understandings of disability. This book does not attempt to provide a comprehensive HIV history because many of the archives it draws from are based in the United States, and New York City in particular. My intention, accordingly, is not to present a cohesive narrative of disability activism but rather to understand many of its components—calling numbers in phone trees, doing the dishes, decorating a hospital ward, hosting HIV Passovers—as inspiring ongoing queer and trans body self-determination. My goal in presenting this limited cross-sampling of archival material is to expand understandings of disability kinship by inviting those we have lost to continue to haunt and to inspire us. I hope, in De La Cruz's words, that *Forget Burial* supports us in "having a good time dealing with" disability, with the disappointments, the fun, and the vulnerabilities of care.

CHAPTER 1

Silence = Undead

VAMPIRES, HIV KINSHIP, AND
COMMUNITIES OF CARE

This chapter begins *Forget Burial*'s project of connecting early HIV caregiving narratives to contemporary disability kinships by drawing inspiration from vampires. Revisiting Octavia Butler's 2005 Afrofuturist novel *Fledgling* reimagines this queer, polyamorous, multiracial, cross-class, rural collective of vampires as also living with HIV. Although the narrative openness of Butler's fiction always invites a broad range of plausible interpretations, this chapter interprets *Fledgling* as a novel about HIV. The vampire metaphor Butler presents is not necessarily an HIV metaphor, yet I regard it as such to link the invention of safer sex by queers in the late 1980s and early 1990s to queer and trans caregiving in the present. Although HIV is never named overtly as "one of humanity's many autoimmune diseases" (69) or as the "retrovirus-like infection" (195) in the novel, Butler's vampires could be an interdependent community of lovers living with HIV. Rather than embodying evil or fear, the Ina vampires might represent an intergenerational HIV community whose practices of exchanging blood and sex lead not to death but to sustaining one another's physical and emotional wellbeing. The novel thus offers metaphorical representations not of curing disability but of generating chosen families for navigating care, negotiating consent, and prison abolition.

HIVAMPIRES

This chapter begins with a close reading of *Fledgling* to provide a model of HIV kinship in response to disability. Building from my analysis of the novel, I then examine issues of sexual consent as they relate to HIV decriminalization and caregiving in the present. Next, I return to histories of safer sex and harm reduction to further connect the production of disability narratives from self-portraits to porn that reframe HIV as a site of care. Reading all these texts together reimagines disability as a site not of shame but of kinship. Reading *Fledgling* as a novel about HIV expands existing narratives of caregiving and disability. Because sci-fi novels, and *Fledgling* in particular, call constant attention to their own fictional status and relative impossibility, this genre actually offers tools for enhancing everyday caregiving practices in tangible ways. *Fledgling* represents concepts rarely associated with care—illness transmission, induction into vampirism, sex across power relations—and grapples with how people support each other through challenging experiences. Reading this vampire metaphor as a metaphor for HIV challenges cultural narratives about illness that create stigma and suffering (Sontag 6; Treichler 11; D. Morris 63; J.W. Jones; Atkins 1989; Davis 37–38; Delany, "Tale of Plagues" 184; Wald 67; Showalter, *Sexual* 4; Bersani 211; Gilman 90; Brandt 5; Hoppe 13). Science fiction builds different worlds through the creation of speculative future possibilities: narrative alters the present by imagining the future differently (Kilgore 127; Ghosh 66). In *Afro-Fabulations: The Queer Drama of Black Life*, Tavia Nyong'o argues that fiction can resist the search for finality and truth that recovering the archive might temptingly offer: "Every attempt at getting closer to the historical truth by way of its archival remains leads to more dead ends and diversions: in the process of establishing the truth, we repeatedly lose the plot" (61). Nyong'o thus argues that the point of archival return might not be recovery at all but can instead provide value in reading fictions precisely because they offer ambivalence, mystery, and indeterminacies that cannot be resolved in linear time, or in the present (202, 7, 47, 51). This methodology of reading novels not to fix history but to "acknowledge the insurrectionary stance taken in the everyday" (Nyong'o 51; Mackenzie 3) considers how HIV might be narrated differently through depictions of care; Butler's vampire metaphor reframes disability not as an individualized body problem but as a collective experience that holds the potential to bring people together. Caregiving in *Fledgling* creates chosen families, HIV community, and alternatives to the prison industrial complex (PIC). Caregiving in this novel, however, does not often look like a reciprocal exchange, as care is given and taken across uneven power dynamics. *Fledgling* sets up contradictions about the caregiving utopia it envisions by portraying interdependence as a community structure that might not always be consensual or even plausible. Butler nevertheless represents fictional responses to disability as motivating kinships and creating interdependence. Because caregiving takes on many different forms from feeding, to housing, to sex, the representation of HIV caregiving in *Fledgling* offers a variety of narrative possibilities for reimagining ongoing queer and trans responses to disability. In analyzing fiction in conjunction with an array of queer caregiving archives and histories of safer sex, this chapter revisits *Fledgling* to link early HIV caregiving activism with current movements for body self-determination.

This chapter is structured around *Fledgling* to connect early safer-sex archives to ongoing queer and trans caregiving and its cultural production. I cut across time between histories of safer sex and contemporary narratives of HIV to link caregiving activism of the past to contemporary disability kinships. The invention of safer sex in the early 1980s can be understood as caregiving: the inception of safer sex as a community-driven initiative to take care of one's partners, one's clients, and oneself through the act of sexual exchange highlights the caregiving potential of sharing information. Like *Fledgling*'s vampires, early HIV archives contain narratives of safer sex as a community-centered, care-driven exchange that supports queer desire and body self-determination into the present. Early grassroots safer sex narratives stand in contrast to biomedical understandings of safer sex that stigmatize individuals by holding them responsible for public health. In taking up these questions of responsibility and consent, *Fledgling*'s fictional narrative also challenges current laws criminalizing the transmission of HIV. Such laws regard HIV transmission as a nonconsensual act requiring disclosure, effectively blaming a seropositive partner for declining to disclose rather than rendering the seronegative partner equally responsible for sexual decision making. Again, such narratives hold individuals and not systemic inequalities responsible for illness and health. Butler's vampires offer a narrative model to reframe sexual practices like HIV nondisclosure that although criminalized can be understood as acts of care. HIV caregiving, *Fledgling* uncovers, can inspire alternatives to incarcerating those who cause harm. Reading HIV novels thus becomes a method for imagining futures without prisons.

FLUID BONDING

As Nina Auerbach argues in *Our Vampires, Ourselves*, the vampire figure evolves alongside our ever-changing cultural preoccupations and fears (6). Since their popularization in the nineteenth century, vampires have become literary signifiers of racial and sexual deviance embodying illnesses as wide ranging as syphilis and tuberculosis (Goddu 133; Patterson 40; N. Nixon 119; Gordon and Hollinger 6; Holmes 180; Gorna 4; M. Jones 154; Hanson 325; Davidson, "Ghosting" 224; Penzenstadler and Birkley 148). *Fledgling*'s narrator Shori, however, radically reinscribes the vampire's traditional function. Shori, a black girl who is also a vampire, builds an intergenerational community of lovers who become each other's "symbionts," becoming "healthier, stronger, and harder to kill" (69) by biting and infecting each other with vampire venom. Although many characters take care of Shori at various points in the plot because she loses her memory and her family in a violent attack, Shori also makes mutual this process of caregiving, creating reciprocal forms of vampire kinship. Because she is experiencing amnesia, Shori must relearn all there is to know about the Ina, the tribe of vampires from which she descends. Shori ridicules the canonical ideas of the vampire as sexual threat or immoral predator, as the Ina "have very little in common with the vampire creatures Bram Stoker described in *Dracula*" (69). Unlike in *Dracula*, the Ina vampires do not drain the life from their human blood sources but rather exchange blood for sexual pleasure and emotional support. The Ina select humans across a wide range of ages, classes, races, and genders to become their symbionts (69), a term used in the novel to suggest the mutuality between humans and vampires who care reciprocally for one another—and physically depend on each other for survival—for the rest of their lives. Once the Ina bite humans, they become linked by blood, forming rural, self-sustaining communities of interdependence. Shori observes how "we don't have to injure the humans we take [blood] from . . . [and] we can't magically convert humans into our kind. We do keep those who join with us healthier, stronger, and harder to kill than they would be without us . . . lengthen[ing] their lives by several decades" (69). The vampiric endeavor of biting thus becomes an act of care by creating resilience in humans and bringing them into Ina kinship structures. Biting is a mutually orgasmic process, a deeply pleasurable exchange of strengthening communal bonds through blood.

While there is no direct indication that Butler's vampires are living with HIV, I nevertheless imagine this text as an HIV narrative by reading this highly sexual swapping of blood as a metaphor for HIV transmission. Rather than regarding this act as undesirable, *Fledgling*'s vampires narrate viral transmission as a pleasurable opportunity for kinship formations: this process of seroconversion (conversion to vampirism) is represented not a moment of regret or of loss but as the precursor to giving and receiving mutual care. Butler's vampires present a family structure through which humans fluid bond eternally to those within their interdependent community. In *Unlimited Intimacy: Reflections on the Subculture of Barebacking*, Tim Dean likewise reframes HIV transmission as opportunity for kinship. Dean rescripts pathologizing narratives to regard seroconversion as creating bloodlines: "One of the most remarkable transformations wrought by the epidemic was this overnight conversion of strangers into relatives, without the usual intermediary stages of friendship or cohabitation" (91). Like Butler's vampire narrative, Dean destigmatizes viral transmission as generative in creating biological ties without heterosexual reproduction (90; Rose 244). He narrates bareback sex as a nontraditional mode of family building that reconceives intimacy as a collective membership process rather than something that transpires between a couple alone (95). The kinship networks that develop among Butler's vampires also offer narratives that challenge HIV stigma by imagining new models of providing care that do not rely on the couple or on an isolated nuclear family unit. *Fledgling* plays with these connective possibilities found in disability, collective caregiving, and queer sex.

In narrating this process of forming kinships through sex, Butler raises challenging questions about caregiving and consent. *Fledgling*'s representations of sex suggest how sexual bonds between lovers may not ever be fully consensual because of the power dynamics that play out within relationships. Obtaining consent is framed as a potential act of caregiving in *Fledgling*, as Shori explores the unity and the tensions between desire and care. In fact, Butler's representation of consent actually creates more feelings of discomfort than feelings of care. This discomfort urges a consideration of how the justice system's attempts to police consent through legal structures fails to effectively support sexual consent in practice. A reading of HIV and consent in this novel is enhanced by the work of crip theorists who reframe disability as a culturally mediated rather than a merely individual phenomenon: crip understandings of illness suggest that reducing stigma and suffering necessitates a narrative shift away from mandating recovery and body norms and toward examining the social contexts in which we experience discomfort (dis-ease?) with embodiments that remind us of our own (human) physical and cognitive limits (Kafer 25; Clare, *Brilliant* 87; McRuer, *Crip* 10; Metzl 3; Lorde 65; Fawaz 137). Butler's consent narratives also do the work of connecting sexual violence to the larger systemic barriers that affect individual bodies. Because narratives create cultural understandings of what consent means and of which subjects are able to give consent and under which circumstances, narrative practices also have the capacity to connect the interpersonal harms caused by sexual violence to wider forces of colonialism, racism, and gender-based oppression: narratives found within fictional texts can expose the larger systemic barriers to consent. The vampire metaphor situates sexual violence as an outcome of institutional and colonial forces including forced migration, criminalization and policing, environmental destruction, and barriers to health-care access and employment (A. Smith 8; Jiwani and Young 911; Simpson 2014; Maynard 67). In contrast to narratives that connect consent and interpersonal harm to systemic violence, legal narratives frame consent as a process that can be addressed (and punished) on a case-by-case, individual level. In *Fledgling*, this individualist punitive criminal paradigm is challenged through Butler's representation of Shori's age. Although Shori appears to be "a child of about ten or eleven" (24), she engages in sexual relationships with a range of adults because as a vampire, she is actually far older than she appears. Any notion of Shori's youth as a legal and ethical barrier to sexual consent is negated by her vampirism. Here Butler plays on generic conventions, suggesting that the novel's essence as science fiction and Shori's status as "not human" (26) override the legal and moral codes governing sexual consent (Lundberg 567). Following Shori's assertion "I didn't have any idea how old I was or why my age should matter" (14), Butler's graphic representation of sex between a (fifty-three-year-old vampire in the body of a) prepubescent child and an adult stranger prompts consideration of how all relationships contain structures of power that influence the process of obtaining consent. In placing consent and power at its center, the novel inverts victim narratives by illustrating how Shori is actually older, stronger, and more experienced than her first symbiont Wright, who has sex with Shori before learning about her vampire age. Sentiments that perhaps Wright is taking advantage of this "elfin little girl" (66) are undermined by the irrefutable power the vampire wields over her human blood source. *Fledgling* reverses the narrative of violence and vulnerability that readers might be expecting (S. Morris 160; Gomez 86; Lundberg 561). Although their relationship is de facto inappropriate, it is nevertheless treated with approval by the romance thread of the novel, creating a sense of uneasiness in witnessing the acts of care that transpire between this couple. It is precisely this uneasiness that compels us to question our predetermined beliefs about the links between creating legal policies and obtaining sexual consent in practice. Instead, Butler's novel uses speculative fiction to raise questions about what sexual consent is beyond legal structures and how it might more holistically be attained as a form of mutual care.

Fledgling fluctuates between representing consent as unattainable and contradictorily rendering negotiations of consent as an expression of care. Consent and care are linked through the narrative's representation of partners overtly navigating the power dynamics and desires between them as humans and vampires. Vampires must take great care in deciding how to appropriately form family with their humans who become communally and biologically tied to their vampires for life by consenting to sex. A lack of care in this process, the narrative reveals, can create much harm in forming families that will erode without informed decision making and trust. Obtaining consent carefully and understanding how difficult (and potentially even impossible) this process can be across power dynamics is one of this novel's fundamental narrative concerns. The first representation of sex in the novel transpires because Shori is injured and needs care from the stranger who picks her up from the side of the road: "I wanted to get into the car with him. I didn't want him to drive away without me. Now that I'd had a few more moments to absorb his scent I realized he smelled . . . really interesting. Also, I didn't want to stop talking to him. I felt almost as hungry for conversation as I was for food" (15). When Shori begins this exchange with Wright, a "broad, and tall" (13) man of twenty-three, dual issues of consent arise concerning Wright's conversion to vampirism and his corresponding sexual desire for Shori, who appears to be prepubescent. When Shori first bites Wright during a struggle in his car, he pulls her onto his lap, prompting her request to let her bite him again. His response, "If I do, what will you let me do?" (18), connotes his sexual attraction to the child in his passenger seat. Shori interprets this display of desire as permission to suck Wright's blood; she observes, "I heard consent in his voice, and I hauled myself up and kissed the side of his neck" (18). Wright's physical desire for Shori prompts his own initiation into vampirism. When Wright brings Shori home, he discerns from what she has told him about her hunting and eating habits that she is not human. When Shori asks, "What if I'm not . . . what would that mean?" (26), Wright's immediate response is to ask Shori to take off her pants. Shori admits, "I don't know enough about myself to say what my age might be or even whether I'm human. But I'm old enough to have sex with you if you want to" (21). Shori's qualifier, "if you want to" (27), is repeated again in the following paragraph, emphasizing that sexual consent is Wright's "reward" (27) for allowing Shori to bite him. These implied links between viral transmission and sexual reward in this exchange are significant because they neither condone nor stigmatize the power imbalance within these negotiations of (informed?) consent. At the basis of these sexual exchanges are Shori's repeated vows of acting from a place of concern as informing her desires. Shori relays—through cuddling, feeding, and sex—her care for her symbionts: "He laughed—a deep, good, sweet sound. By touch and scent I found the large, tempting artery. I bit him, took his blood, and rode his leg as he convulsed and shouted" (198). For Shori, the exchange of blood and sex with humans is an act of caregiving in the sense that vampire venom provides pleasure and healing but also because it needs to be administered *carefully*. As such, sex is an act that Shori approaches quite judiciously, always cautious not to take more than she needs from each symbiont. This care is demonstrated through her labor of healing, pleasuring, and verbally obtaining consent from the humans she invites into her family. Upon receiving consent, however, Shori realizes that the hastiness with which it is given to her is surprising. For instance, upon inviting her second symbiont, Theodora, to come live in her communal arrangement, Shori considers, "I had been careful to let her make up her own mind, and I had believed she would come with me, but not so quickly" (98). Consent is therefore rendered as a precursor to sex (and biting) that must be constantly renegotiated as an ongoing reciprocal caregiving exchange in support of self-determination. It is through this negotiation process that *Fledgling* addresses the wider cultural forces within which these negotiations operate.

Fledgling takes up difficult questions of power and consent to show how even in situations when consent cannot freely be given, it must still be strived for on an ongoing basis to address the structural inequalities that make consent difficult to achieve interpersonally. As Shori is initially unable to disclose her vampire identity to Wright, the desire that transpires between them is at once consensual and upsetting due to their multitude of power imbalances. Butler builds the reader's enthusiasm as well as discomfort in response to Shori's ability to manipulate humans through sex, as the control she wields over her partners is both disturbing and exciting for all parties. Humans may initially walk away from their Ina symbionts, but the narrative poses a trap for readers to ponder, as although it is plausible to wean from the immense pleasures of vampire venom, the psychic and physical consequences of separation are excruciating, especially once "deeply attached to the source of the substance" (79). Once separated from their Ina partners, humans "die unless another one of us is able to take them over" (80). The narrative thereby suggests that although being coerced into and later addicted to vampirism might never be fully consensual, the results of remaining in community with vampires might also never be fully adverse. This tension points to the importance of care in this process of obtaining consent and in navigating nondisclosure. The desire to not disclose one's status (as a vampire) is respected as a form of body self-determination; protecting this choice to not disclose can therefore also be read as an act of caregiving even if this act of nondisclosure is by definition nonconsensual. Obtaining consent on the one hand and supporting nondisclosure on the other, are both exchanges in the narrative that are navigated with care. However, the safety and sovereignty of the subjects in these relationships is always overdetermined not merely by the kindness with which individuals treat one another but also by the larger structural forces that shape cultural narratives of vampirism and thereby Ina practice.

By positioning this erotic coercion and addiction as factors that are not necessarily negative, even for the individual who is addicted or coerced, Butler complicates understandings of consent and desire as they relate to the transmission of HIV. In the context of tenacious laws criminalizing HIV transmission on the grounds of sexual nonconsent (Duke, "Consent" 2015; Symington 9), this novel raises timely questions about how these laws do not deter sexual violence but ultimately create more harm and racism, as the majority of people prosecuted under HIV nondisclosure laws are also facing antiblack and colonial violence from within the justice system (Symington 9; Velasquez-Potts 105; Vowel 49, 36). As scholars have shown, enforcing the disclosure of one's HIV status prior to having sex can increase risk of violence and isolation for people living with HIV, disproportionately affecting those in already vulnerable power dynamics, who already face gender-based, colonial, and racist violence (Velasquez-Potts 107; Symington 9; Duke, "Consent"; McClelland and Whitbread 92; PASAN 63). Butler's larger corpus includes works like *Dawn* (1987), "Bloodchild" (1996), *Clay's Ark* (1984), and *Wild Seed* (1980), which also play centrally with whether the loss of bodily control that results from sex, interdependence, and other pleasure-driven activities can ever be fully consensual (Vint 59; Alaimo 130). In *Dawn*, the Oankali aliens expand the human Lilith's sexual practices, urging her to incorporate multiple partners at once and to have sexual relationships with those whose gender identities cannot be labeled as either female or male. These novel forms of sexuality are highly pleasurable to Lilith, yet she continually fears the implications of having her sexual capacities extended "beyond ordinary human experience" (161). In spite of the ambiguity of consent across Butler's writing, novels including *Wild Seed* resolve by pointing to the undesirable alternative of a life without intimacy and connection (and without the accompanying physical risks that invariably follow). Like Butler's fiction, Cohen and Livingston argue that HIV makes apparent the dangers that occur "when we live together" but that such dangers reveal the simultaneous "impossibility of living alone" (40); Cohen and Livingston therefore read "AIDS" as signifying the interdependence of bodies, reminding us how the acronym "doubles the word 'aids' in the sense of assists, helps, supports, succors" (41). By criminalizing people living with HIV for transmitting the virus, even when their seronegative partners consent to the possibility of sexual infection (Symington 9), such laws demonstrate an inability to imagine that humans would ever consent to hosting a virus that could mark our bodies as diseased, alien, dependent, addicted, as pleasurable, or as falling outside of medical norms (Bailey 218, 222). Denying the possibility that humans might actually desire to engage in risky sex or illegal substance use ignores the complexity of risk and disability taken up within Butler's fiction. *Fledgling* thus presents the vampire metaphor to challenge narratives that we must all strive to be normal and healthy rather than taking power in being disabled or different. As fiction, the novel creates a conceptual opportunity to challenge this cultural narrative of imperative normalcy and health, as Butler's vampire metaphor imagines an interdependent HIV community whose practices of exchanging blood and sex lead not to harm but to kinship.

WE'RE GOING TO CARE FOR PEOPLE

This next section extends out of Butler's vampire narrative to consider how early HIV archives support disability kinships in the present. In imagining disability not as cause for shame but as motivating interdependence, a return to archival narratives of HIV links these caregiving legacies to ongoing disability movements. In an ACT UP Oral History Project interview, lesbian filmmaker and ACT UP/New York member Jean Carlomusto discusses how narratives of HIV caregiving were initially constructed as oppositional to frontline work. Carlomusto's interview pinpoints the creation of an unnecessary narrative division between caregiving and civil disobedience in New York City in the late 1980s:

> It was a contest for who was going to control the discourse around AIDS. Was it going to be in an increasingly professional model, like "We're going to care for people. We're going to set up this whole professional organization to manage the care and advocacy of people living with AIDS," which was the GMHC model. Or was it going to be, "The rules are fucked and nothing's going to change until we get out there and we change them, and we advocate." So really the two messages should have been complementary and not competitive, because there was a need to have an organization that was managing care for people with AIDS, because the changes did not happen automatically. And GMHC lessened the suffering, and continues to lessen the suffering of people with AIDS. But at the same time, without ACT UP there would be no changing of society. (40)

As Carlomusto's interview reveals, these two seemingly opposing objectives of providing care and demanding change are most effective in combination. Caregiving and frontline activism need not be understood as mutually exclusive (Brier 170; McRuer, "Disability" 58; Crimp et al. 128; Spade 33; Hollibaugh 138; Gould 339). ACT UP/New York activist, scholar, and artist Debra Levine also reflects on ACT UP's mutual practice of activism and care: "In demonstrations organized by affinity, care is local, specific, imaginative, and creative" (22; Bauer 20). This process of collaboration characteristic of affinity groups generates queer familial bonds that are both artistic and sexual, as Levine explains: "Acting in affinity often felt good" (87): "We . . . consciously adapted the forms of resistance we performed so well on the street to the site of the hospital room" (112). The community that "happens" (28) from such acts of care, Levine asserts, "serves as a critique of what is present" (28). Returning now to these affinity narratives connects these earlier critiques of "what is present" to the ongoing interventions of contemporary queer and trans caregiving.

Like the queer kinds of care exchanged by Butler's vampires, HIV activism offers a model of caregiving in response to state neglect that supports bodies that fail to participate in capitalist exchange. Rather than offer a type of care to be simply adopted within or outside of the existing state, these histories of HIV kinship serve to challenge the state itself for creating barriers to mutual support. The early HIV archive contains narratives of disability as inspiring a critique of capitalism, racism, and colonialism that can be reanimated in the present. The NYPL archive, for instance, houses the unpublished diaries of Bradley Ball, who served as the first recording secretary of ACT UP. Ball's diaries and letters chart his own shifting perspectives about state systems through his experience of living with HIV. Ball draws from bell hooks's observation that "as more middle class white women lose status and enter the ranks of the poor, they may find it necessary to criticize capitalism. . . . Hard times have a remarkable way of opening your eyes." As Ball reflects in an entry from 1990, "Certainly my abrupt slide from white-collar administrator to unemployed, to unemployable, to suicidally depressed, to welfare recipient, to disability recipient intensified my radical orientation from liberal reformist to revolutionary anarchist." Revisiting these early HIV archives continues to create care networks that transform rather than rely on existing systems to provide mutual aid. HIV archives are thus foundational to contemporary acts of forming queer and trans chosen family in response to systems that create barriers to access and to affinity.

Toward resisting narratives of undesirability and of body shame, these HIV archives can be connected to ongoing queer caregiving kinships. Early HIV narratives that link caregiving, activism, and sex can be read as informing the contemporary work of Toronto-based academic and "femmegimp" (femme, queer, crip) porn star Loree Erickson. Like Butler's vampires and the affinity archives of ACT UP, Erickson's 2006 pornographic film *Want* shares with viewers Erick-

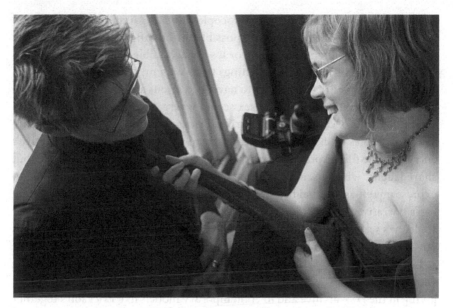

Figure 1.1. Loree Erickson takes care of her care collective's needs in her femmegimp porn *Want* (2006). Courtesy of Loree Ericson. Photo credit: David Findley.

son's "personal care needs" that include assistance with daily tasks but also include queer and trans sex (see fig. 1.1). Porn becomes a medium through which to value disabled bodies for their teachings on "touch, dependency, and vulnerability" (Erickson, "Revealing" 44; Fawaz 149). The film simultaneously presents sexual partners caring for each other's desires alongside the anticapitalist care collectives that fulfill the basic attendant care needs of the film's star. Pornographic representation links these two forms of care that are frequently (mis) represented as antithetical. Although the film uses transitions like title screens and musical cues to separate the sex scenes between Erickson and her costar from the scenes of daily assistance from her care collective, presenting them together in the same film demonstrates how the daily care she receives from her collective supports her not only with basic tasks but with expressing her basic needs. Another title screen introducing the care collective discusses the political context of its creation: "This collective started in response to the inadequacy of public funding for personal care and staffing difficulties due to the homophobia of many of the paid personal attendants. I have been extremely fortunate to meet my care needs in this way." As narratives of HIV organizing demonstrate, the failure of the state to provide adequate care prompts not only activism to change state systems but also organizing to take care back at a community level. It is Erickson's chosen family and not the state that will get her what she wants: "I want to be recognized as a good friend but also as a good fuck. I'm sick of being seen as incompetent, childlike, and inspirational, simply because the environment wasn't constructed with people who have disabilities in mind. I'm tired of waiting for the next bus and possibly the bus after that one because the lift on this one is either not working or it's not accessible to begin with. And by the way, I can think of a lot better things to do with my time." The visuals then cut from scenes of Erickson trying to navigate various accessibility barriers like public transportation back to the sex scenes where moaning and laughter represent the kinds of care that characterizes Erickson as building sites of pleasure to counter "sites of shame" (42). A title screen preempting the care collective's entry into the film expresses, "I not only receive care based on mutual aid, but share laughs, wisdoms, and sorrows. [The care collective] also enables me to express myself as a sexual being without fear of abuse or denial of care." Erickson's narrative exposes that like caring for someone's daily needs, caring for someone's sexual wants (as porn) exposes the power of interdependence as based on "the mutuality of these caring relationships . . . contribut[ing] to new ways of being-in-the-world-with-others" (45). Like the activism of ACT UP and the vampire communities of *Fledgling*, the kinds of kinships that form out of caregiving in the HIV archive and in contemporary models like Erickson's together bridge early responses to HIV with ongoing disability kinships.

It is thus generative to read Erickson's contemporary queer and trans care collective not as an isolated historical moment but as part of the ongoing legacy of early HIV caregiving. For instance, the parallel representation of both attendant care and porn in Erickson's work might be interpreted as controversial in relationship to the abuses and power imbalances that disabled people have survived when relying on others for care; however, in reading this narrative in connection to histories of HIV caregiving, Erickson's work can be understood as productively negotiating sexual desire and pleasure as part of and not as antithetical to caregiving. Erickson's representation of disability as sexy and as forming queer and trans kinships continues to make space for sexual desire and chosen family formation to coexist alongside—and because of—the vulnerabilities of exchanging care. Like Butler's vampire fiction, Erickson does not avoid these issues of consent but directly represents sex as an opportunity to investigate power relationships outside of state-supported systems. Rather than rely on a separation between care and sex as an antidote to these potential power imbalances, Erickson creates porn in order to represent how power and consent are negotiated through collective caregiving when one's care team is created "from my community." As such, her work can be linked to Butler's fiction and to the queer and trans kinships formed in early responses to HIV that integrate rather than attempt to eliminate the connections between the exchange of power and the exchange of care.

Another contemporary artist whose work reframes negotiations of power and consent as an exchange of care is that of Mikiki (who identifies as a mixed white/indigenous person of Mi'kmaq, Acadian, and Irish heritage), a queer video and

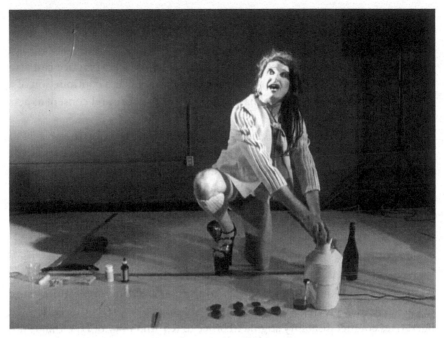

Figure 1.2. Mikiki performs *On the Department of Experimental Medicine* (2005–2011) at Trigger Festival, Toronto (2008). Courtesy of the artist.

performance artist and sexual health educator who is also based in Toronto (see fig. 1.2). Like Butler's vampire narrative, Mikiki's work represents the kinships formed in response to HIV. Through the genre of personal narrative, Mikiki discusses their commitment to building the HIV community, addressing care explicitly for a queer and trans readership. In an interview for the queer art journal *No More Potlucks*, Mikiki discusses their work as an HIV artist and peer outreach worker before they seroconverted. This long-standing practice of HIV activism, Mikiki shares, informed their experience of building community to address HIV stigma and to complicate narratives of blame and harm underwriting narratives of HIV transmission. Mikiki stages performances to raise questions of self-determination and consent via their own bodily fluids. One such performance features an enormous self-made public glory hole whose exterior reads, "MIKIKI is inside this box / One day/night only/ Saturday May 25th 2007/ come inside/ and go/ down in a blaze of/ GLORY HOLE/ this is a performance." In a recording from this event, *These Conversations, But with People We're Hot For*, the camera documents Mikiki close-up from inside the box. Mikiki discusses with a visitor to the box that this performance makes space to stage negotiations for gaining pleasure through public sexual cultures without conceding to the desires of others that run counter to one's own needs. Mikiki shows that in the glory hole performance, these conversations with friends became grounds for envisioning renewed community accountability and support: "And then we got to kiss through that little hole." Mikiki's performance connects community building to discussions of consent, expanding the definition of care as a process of supporting sexual self-determination. Mikiki's art practice can also be read as extending early HIV activism into the present, as a continuation of a longer queer and trans lineage of navigating sexual pleasure and consent as acts of care.

Mikiki's art-based narratives extend early HIV narratives into the present to redefine disability not as a site of shame but as restoring sexual agency to bodies marked as different. Mikiki's work also raises the very questions of responsibility and power that Shori considers fictionally in learning about vampires. While Butler's vampires trouble the possibility of obtaining consent outside of preset power relationships, Mikiki's performances offer a space for consensual negotiations of sexual pleasure for people living with HIV. As in Butler's novel, Mikiki's work reframes sexual risk as holding the potential for creating care rather than equating HIV transmission with narratives of harm. The differences in genre between Mikiki's art-based practice and Butler's fiction reflect the range of narrative strategies that can disrupt body shaming by representing care. Such narratives counter disability stigma in order to tell "the story of HIV that is not spoken of." In contrast to the gothic fantasies of Butler's fiction—a genre that relies on metaphor to share the experience of stigma—Mikiki's writing draws on sincerity and on realism to reframe HIV community as one of mutual care. Demonstrating a candidness central also to Erickson's porn, Mikiki again uses the first person to represent "people making their own decisions . . . and having them backfire. And finding ways of continuing their relationships through that. And acknowledging that we make decisions, and we're ok with them at the time, but we can't see the future." In narrating how intimate relationships are built through the process of disclosing one's status, Mikiki like Butler reimagines seroconverting as a process of forming disability kinships. In negotiating sexual desires and risks, Mikiki's work figures nonconforming bodies as beautiful, messy, and tenacious, creating spaces of mutual care that, in Erickson's words, "move to a place where disabled people and our bodies are appreciated and wanted, not in spite of our differences, but because of them" (46). These contemporary movements for queer and trans body self-determination can be linked back to early HIV archives via these conversations of disclosure and consent. Navigating and supporting decision making about disclosure can be read as on ongoing act of care, even when a partner self-determines not to disclose, and even when the process of obtaining consent is overdetermined by larger power structures and forms of anti-queer and gender-based violence that Mikiki's art calls into focus.

How we narrate HIV in the present is also connected to how we continue to preserve and recirculate stories of HIV's caregiving histories. Visual AIDS curator and artist Ajamu investigates this process by interviewing fourteen young activists of color about their work as it connects to objects and the archiving process. In a 2016 video portrait with Ajamu, New York City–based multidisciplinary artist Kia LaBeija discusses her experience of building HIV community through her art and activism: "There's no community for children born with the HIV virus so it's been a really incredible journey figuring it out." LaBeija discusses the work of Visual AIDS in archiving the contributions of people who "are not here anymore" as well as showcasing the work of living artists. She considers the impact of Visual AIDS: "[It's a] platform to be an artist, to be a working artist, and to share my story and experiences with a broader audience has been really incredibly impactful for me so I think it's very very important to archive the work that's been made by people living with HIV and people that are making work around it because it's that constant conversation, because art is a conversation . . . it's a way to keep talking about it" ("Ajamu's"). LaBeija's self-portraits initiate such conversations by presenting the artist within a series of intimate domestic spaces—bathrooms, boudoirs, bedroom floors—that invite the viewer to peer in from a distance in an act of admiring LaBeija's black, Native American, Filipino, queer female body living with HIV. Many of LaBeija's self-portraits feature domestic life but one image from the clinic spotlights the seated artist, clad in red crinoline and sequins, a single white rose on her lap, gazing straight into the viewer's eyes as her blood is taken by a white man in a suit. This self-portrait, *Eleven*, premiered on the eleventh anniversary of her mother's passing (*Eleven* is also featured on *Forget Burial*'s cover). In an interview with Jasmin Hernandez, LaBeija discusses how the man in the suit is indeed her doctor, and he is indeed drawing her blood for the portrait. She also reveals that the dress she is wearing was her prom dress, a symbol of her survival because she was "a child who was expected to die before the age of 7." "This is my interpretation of how I see myself every time I sit on that slab," shares LaBeija, linking glamour to the clinic and to the bodies who frequent it. In framing her own process of resilience, LaBeija creates a representation of women living with HIV as one of beauty: "I wanted to express that women and girls who live with the virus are beautiful beyond belief and that no matter what society says, we are sexy and we deserve love. I have thought long and hard about the phrase 'beauty lies within,' people say 'its not what's on the outside, but what is on the inside that counts.' What happens when the world tells you that your insides are considered a deadly weapon?" (Hernandez) While Erickson expands cultures of desirability through film, LaBeija's photography counters the desexualization of disabled bodies using self-portraiture: "I also think it's so important for women living with HIV to feel sexy. I think we need to be reminded that we too can have desires and live fulfilling sex lives" (*Duets* 42). In her artist's statement on the Visual AIDS website, the portrait is given the dedication "For my Mother" and the statement itself presents a poetic depiction of the work. LaBeija connects life to death, elegizing her mother through the process of remembering: "When she died, I cried just as hard as the day I met her." In *Eleven*, the clinic becomes a memorial place: "Every time he takes my blood I think of her, because we share it. Because she has sat here on this same table. And because I am the last piece of her left in this world." LaBeija then signs the statement: "Love, / Your daughter." In addressing her mother's ghost, LaBeija visually captures the presence her mother's absence holds in her life, inviting the viewer to take part in this display of care.

LaBeija's portraits create feelings of voyeuristic inappropriateness alongside portraiture's invitation to look in, presenting a haunting beauty that conjures the clinic but inverts the act of staring back toward the viewer. The rich colors and theatrical vibrancy characteristic of LaBeija's portraiture speak back to the narrative desexualization of women living with HIV, challenging the viewer to acknowledge preconceptions about medicalized bodies and the objects that surround them (Mitchell and Whitbread 2011; Schulman, "Dear" 118). Nyong'o reads this portrait as a performance of blackness that holds the potential to "rearrange our perceptions of chronology, time, and temporality" (4) through LaBeija's addressing "us, here in the future, without being able to know how she has changed us" (4). In "mingling what was with what might have been" (7), Nyong'o identifies LaBeija's performance as offering future "possibilities outside our present terms of order" (6). When asked about the archival objects that are important to her work, LaBeija reflects,

> There's one that definitely speaks out to me. . . . Jessica Lynn Whitbread . . . started a project called *Tea Time*. The *Tea Time* project is incredible because it brings together positive women from anywhere she goes travelling whether it's for conference or a lecture or an exhibition and she brings together women living with HIV for a tea party. And at the tea party she asks everybody to bring a teacup and a letter for an exchange for another woman living with HIV. The letter can be . . . anything you want it to be. And you bring a teacup. So I feel like when I first went to this tea party with Jessica that was the first time I started to connect with women because after losing my Mom I was just completely cut off from anything. And so I think that teacup that I have and I hold and has a very special place in my house is something that is very special to me in being this kind of marker of the beginning of my journey. That would be the most important, well, the most special thing—physical object—that I hold. (LaBeija)

LaBeija links the archiving process to the sustenance of kinship ties. HIV community, her work illustrates, is documented through portraits, teacups, and other ephemera that connect archives from the 1980s and 1990s to emerging art and activisms today. In conversation with Julie Tolentino, LaBeija reflects, "In ballroom, the idea of being an icon or legend is key because an icon can never die. I think a lot of these photos are my way of creating my own immortality, or consistently being in conversation with people for the rest of time" (*Duets* 35). The early caregiving legacies of HIV can be preserved by these objects and the narratives through which we remember them. In discussing with LeBeija the importance of sexual representations of women living with HIV, Tolentino recalls how in 1993, "Cynthia Madansky and I wrote the *Safer Sex Handbook for Lesbians* with Gay Men's Health Crisis and Lesbian AIDS Project, and it was sexy! We offered grassroots distribution through our networks to share information about HIV awareness and how pleasure and sex defines much of who we are and how we communicate. I think I have a few packets in my files. I'll give you one—there are gloves and a condom still inside them, but they are a bit dusty now" (42). The intergenerational collaborations between Tolentino and LaBeija bring this dusty latex and its caregiving histories into the present. The section that follows returns to archives of the communities that formed through the process of inventing safer sex. Recalling these narratives draws inspiration from LaBeija's project of continuing to preserve and to create objects that continue to redefine disability.

Harshly Criticized when We First Proposed It

This section revisits the HIV archives of the 1980s and 1990s to connect this contemporary work of disability artists to early narratives of queers inventing safer sex in order to take care of themselves and their partners (Schulman, *My American History* 113; Patton, "Resistance and the Erotic" 70; Carlomusto, "Sex"; Berkowitz 2). Connecting past and present brings narratives of early HIV prevention together with ongoing queer and trans movements for caregiving in response to disability. As with the narrative model of Butler's vampires, early HIV communities formed in response to sexual stigma. Returning to these narratives can continue to reframe disability as an opportunity for queer and trans kinship formations into the present. During the early 1980s, public health messages about the dangers of promiscuity and the need for abstinence were challenged by queer community members including sex workers and health-care practitioners who regarded caregiving as necessitating access to information (Patton, *Globalizing* 66; Gould 77; Carlomusto, *Sex*). Queers recognized from visits to their own doctors—who wore latex gloves while examining them—that latex barrier use could be effectively promoted at a grassroots, community-specific level (Berkowitz 140; Ma 26). In 1982, HIV activist and sex worker Richard Berkowitz created, with Michael Callen and their doctor Joseph Sonnabend, one of the first-ever educational safer-sex publications, *How to Have Sex in an Epidemic: One Approach*. Berkowitz recalls piloting the use of latex barriers during a paid BDSM (Bondage and Discipline, Dominance and Submission, Sadism and Masochism) scene with his client as an act that felt "safe, protective, and caring" (140). Inventing safer sex as a caregiving response to HIV, queer and trans communities began their own advocacy work for access to sex education (Brier 1; Pearl, *AIDS Literature* 64). Creating and sharing medical information therefore became a form of care, and the distribution of this knowledge happened on a community level, bringing together lovers, professionals, and friends through this process of creating access to sex education. Safer sex became a tool for supporting bodily autonomy around sexual decision making, risk taking, and access to pleasure (Gould 66; Race 7).

Safer sex archives preserve these responses to state violence by narrating this antiracist caregiving labor as it extends into the present. Safer sex archives contain narratives of people of color building HIV kinships within their own communities to address gaps created by white-dominated prevention campaigns. In creating communities in response to disability, these grassroots initiatives address racism and medical neglect by providing safer-sex information. Like the forms of community care imagined through Butler's fiction, documentary narrative provides a tool through which to archive and now revisit the continued impact of this process of antiracist community building in response to HIV. In Ellen Spiro's 1989 video *DiAna's Hair Ego*, documentary film brings viewers into the intimate space of DiAna DiAna's hair salon in Columbia, South Carolina. The film informs viewers how beginning in 1986, DiAna provides condoms and information in her salon in response to systemic barriers to accessing HIV education in black Southern communities. DiAna shares information while styling clients' hair, a daily act of caregiving performed through intimate conversational exchange. DiAna also provides a range of safer-sex materials and events in her salon including movie screenings, a telephone hotline, kids' programming, sex toy parties, and musical performances (some of which are captured by the documentary) (Spiro, *DiAna's Hair Ego*; Juhasz, *AIDS TV* 152; DiAna, *Curlers* 13). The limits of capitalism in supporting these exchanges are also evidenced by the lack of external or state resources with which DiAna runs this programming, in her own house. The caregiving resources created and exchanged in DiAna's home and community include ASL (American Sign Language) translations and other tools for increasing the materials' accessibility. Spiro documents how for the creation of one resource, DiAna and her partner Bambi Sumpter film questions that local children have about HIV, questions that Sumpter identifies as quite "graphic." DiAna recalls that students in the third grade were asking the same questions as students in college, demonstrating that HIV education was not taking place, and that the work DiAna and Sumpter were undertaking was filling a critical gap (DiAna, "DiAna's"). At an HIV/AIDS lecture series presentation at Concordia University in 2013, DiAna discusses the barriers she faced in completing this caregiving work. She attests that although she was sustained by the encouragement and support from members of her community, government administrators consistently blocked her from accessing grants and funding. DiAna was forced to fund the South Carolina AIDS Education Network out of pocket until she could no longer afford to provide additional services beyond condom and information distribution within the salon itself. Spiro's film documents how the Department of Environmental Control attempted to "misinterpret" the organization's educational material and "use it against [the organization]." The documentary thus witnesses how institutional racism blocks grassroots education taking place within black communities. "I'm almost back where I started," DiAna states in 2013; "from what I can see, it hasn't changed that much from 1986." Despite the state's continued blocking of community care, DiAna's work nevertheless offers a model for resisting institutional racism through acts of information sharing. DiAna's ongoing work can inspire us to continue to address these barriers to sex education.

Understanding the invention of safer sex as a practice of care exposes how latex barrier use from its invention was a collective effort to support sexual expression rather than an individual onus to safeguard public health. As Allan Brandt identified as early as 1985, because an individual's behavior is subject to complex psychological forces as well as social and economic pressures, the possibility of abrupt individual behavioral modification as a public health measure is untenable (186). Julia Epstein identifies the fallacy of blaming an individual's viral transmission instead of social conditions and resource allocation for the incidence of illness (J. Epstein, *Altered* 171; Dean 61; Brandt 161; Hoppe 44; Jordan-Zachery 121). Rather than being held responsible for public health, individuals could be understood through this safer-sex archive as caring for their kin and their communities' survival, a concept Gregory Tomso identifies as expanding beyond physical survival alone (104). In linking the invention of safer sex to disability caregiving in the present, these personal and communal decisions around self-care (or not) can be understood as ongoing expressions of queer and trans body self-determination.

This link between early HIV and contemporary narratives of mutual care, for instance, is central to Scott Treleavan's 2013 *PosterVirus* poster, which in stark black and white imagery relays the message, "Look after each other." In his artist's statement, Treleavan argues, "Queers, especially younger ones, seem to be fatigued when it comes to AIDS awareness, and I think this is largely due to the awful, exclusionary push towards 'normalizing' queer culture. The message, to look after each other, is always worth reiterating. We've always watched out for one another when no one else would. And this message is becoming more important than ever." Treleavan's work thus connects the anticapitalist and antinormative underpinnings of early HIV activism to ongoing queer and trans caregiving. Another contemporary queer and trans artistic collaboration responding to the ongoing narrative meanings of latex barrier use is that of Morgan M. Page's poster for *PosterVirus*, created in collaboration with LA-based interdisciplinary artist Onya Hogan-Finlay. The poster was inspired by a conversation between

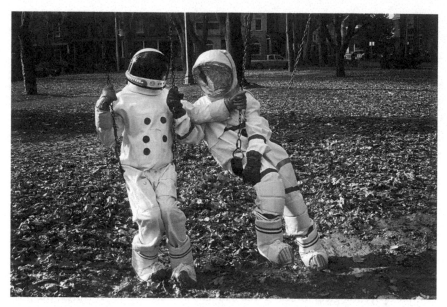

Figure 1.3. Jessica Whitbread and Morgan M. Page share a tender moment on the swing set. Courtesy of Jessica Whitbread and Morgan M. Page. Photo credit: Tania Anderson.

Page and Whitbread about how Whitbread once needed to tell a date, "I don't need to wear a spacesuit to fuck you." The project thus considers "the intersection of the criminalization of HIV non-disclosure, the 'safer sex industrial complex,' and queer women's sexualities" (Whitbread, "Space Dates"). The poster features lesbian astronaut Sally Ride scissoring with a full-armored space suit in a "retro-futuristic feminist landscape." This poster also expands into Whitbread and Page's corresponding *Space Dates* video and photo series of two serodiscordant dykes making out in full astronaut attire in broad daylight on the streets of Toronto (see fig. 1.3). The project invites viewers to appreciate the "cute dates" this pair undertakes via their attempts "to have so-safe-you-can't-even-feel-it sex." Reading this work alongside early HIV archives uncovers how narratives of disability stigma have shifted the meanings of latex barrier use from its inception in the 1980s into the present. *Space Dates* demonstrates how safer sex changes meanings when it moves out of the community-based cultures of care wherein it was invented and into biomedical models that stigmatize seroconversion through individual narratives of maintaining public health. *Space Dates* also revisits historical lesbian iconographies to include trans lesbians. In addressing this shift in the meanings of barrier use for lesbians across time, *Space Dates* invokes cis and trans women's kinships and sexual caregiving practices toward destigmatizing disability in support of queer and trans body self-determination.

Revisiting these archives of safer sex in connection to *Fledgling* also reimagines how fulfilling one's sexual desires and navigating power dynamics can be narrated as an act of caregiving. *Fledgling*'s narrative depicts sex as inherently risky and thus prompting extra compassion for all parties involved. Shori, for instance, presents herself as a caregiver, not just in giving and taking pleasure but in navigating a balance between herself and her symbionts. Shori must take care not to focus too much sexual attention on any one human, as too much biting can cause her symbionts harm in spite of the pleasure experienced in the moment of the exchange. Resisting codependency in favor of a more "mutualistic" (129) model, Shori must "take blood from several symbionts instead of draining one person until [she] kill[s] him" (90). The interest and joy Shori experiences in building an interdependent family of multiple partners creates painful jealousy in Wright, who regards additional partners as threats. Shori, however, reframes Wright's jealousy as that which will "hurt the family" (164), and Shori must demonstrate for Wright how the Ina create kinships to meet the needs of all family members by creating an interconnected community structure. In an interview with Marilyn Mehaffy and AnaLouise Keating, Butler herself asserts, "I always automatically create community. This has to do with the way I've lived. . . . My own feeling is that human beings need to live that way and we too often don't" (51). Interdependence, "biodiversity" (Murray and Bauman xviii), and caregiving bonds between very different individuals (vampire and human) are what support Shori and her people's survival. As Ann Folwell Stanford observes of Butler's EARTHSEED series, "it is community and not individualism that ultimately makes survival possible" (217). The invention of safer sex as a communal process likewise links survival to desire as acts of care. The HIV kinships of Butler's vampires suggest that sexual desire is most effectively realized if sexual practices are defined with openness and curiosity—deciding "how to take my pleasure with you" (254) instead of remaining "lonely but safe" (143). Safety involves a caregiving negotiation between breaking isolation and acknowledging the power dynamics and risks inherent in connecting with (the fluids) of others. Butler's vampire narrative therefore frames care as necessitating kinship, and kinship among vampires cannot be established without the risky, interdependent, and trauma-informed process of biting, fluid-swapping, and sex (Lundberg 577). The fictional representation of this narrative process in *Fledgling* informs a return to this intricate negotiation of pleasure and risk within early archives of HIV.

HIV archives navigate this complex interplay of and tension between desire and risk. The narratives and community debates found within these archives reframe safer sex as a potentially connective experience. These narratives are important because they shape this discussion itself—this navigating how to provide care in response to disability—as the relational outcome of negotiating sex. While *Fledgling* presents a fictional narrative of how to navigate desire in spite of its physical and emotional risks, the autobiographical narratives in the HIV archives discuss the inception of safer sex as fraught with controversies over what taking care in response to disability might look like. Carlomusto revisits these controversies in her 2009 documentary *Sex in an Epidemic*, which traces the state's blocking of safer-sex initiatives in the 1980s when they were invented by queers, as well as the hotbed of community deliberations their invention provoked (Carlomusto 2009; Wein 2008). *Surviving AIDS*, the 1990 autobiography of community organizer and queer singer Callen, who coauthored *How to Have Sex in an Epidemic: One Approach* with Berkowitz and well as authoring *Surviving and Thriving with AIDS*, also examines the process of inventing of safe(r) sex. Callen recalls, "Although 'avoiding the exchange of potentially infectious bodily fluids' has now become the accepted standard of HIV/AIDS risk reduction, we were harshly criticized—especially by the Gay Men's Health Crisis (GMHC)—when we first proposed it" (Callen, *Surviving AIDS* 7). Such debates over the creation and practice of safer sex are also documented in a GMHC Oral History interview with Larry Mass, which resides in the New York Public Library (NYPL) archives on a VHS tape. The author of a critical body of the emerging literature on HIV, Mass produced some of the earliest HIV journalism published in the gay newspaper *The New York Native*. A gay physician and HIV activist, Mass worked to reenvision how a wide range of queer sex acts could be practiced without the transmission of HIV. In the oral history interview, Mass recalls how in the early 1980s, many gay men were deeply concerned that fears of viral transmission would undermine the revolutionary work of gay men in the 1970s who advocated for nonmonogamous, sex-positive relationship configurations and public sexual expressions. Mass worked with other members of the gay community to protect what he views as "non-negotiable" advances in queer life: "I was not willing to retreat . . . from my belief in the greater values of the sexual revolution. And I fought very hard early on in the epidemic to maintain those values and withhold them." As HIV activist and theorist Jennifer Brier identifies, the important historical contexts and sexual politics underlying these debates among queer community organizers were lost to reductive biomedical messages about condom use and illness transmission that replaced these holistic discussions of "the meaning of gay liberation" (44). These early safer-sex debates also spotlighted a political division between queers defending nonconformist public sexual cultures and those who advocated for a politics of "respectability" (Gould 75; 60; 71). HIV continues to be cited into the present as justification for championing normative relationship models over nonconforming sexual expressions (Castiglia and Reed 48; Jordan-Zachery 122). As David Román identifies in his 2006 reading of the 1990 HIV film *Longtime Companion*, revisiting HIV narratives in the present allows us to gain new perspectives about queer survival.

In reflecting on these respectability narratives in our contemporary moment in relationship to pre-exposure prophylaxis (PrEP), Nathan Lee and Carlos Motta also return to the 1980s and safer-sex history to consider political positions like Crimp's "arguing on behalf of promiscuity *as* a survival strategy." Lee and Motta also link PrEP to histories of feminism and birth control, as well as queer and trans organizing, to discuss constructions of biomedicine in making sex "natural" or "denaturalized" through cultural and medical storytelling. Lee and Motta draw on the initial invention of safer sex to connect PrEP's cultural narratives to ongoing histories of queers "loving and taking care of each other." This approaching of PrEP discourse from a place of love and care, Lee and Motta's work argues, requires intersectionally critiquing the medical industrial complex and broader capitalist systems that make Truvada inaccessible to many in the United States and transnationally (Lee and Motta; Hoppe 65). Their reading of PrEP narratives demonstrates how discourses about disability normalize the suffering of nonwhite subjects through narratives that frame certain bodies as deserving access to health and others as necessarily experiencing debility. As Puar argues, narratives of disability create a privileged identity for those who have (or are framed as holding the right to have) medical access by normalizing the harm experienced by subjects facing transnational structural barriers to care under neoliberalism, settler colonialism, and militarization (*Right to Maim* xv). Jih-Fei Cheng's work traces this process in relation to PrEP: "The increased focus on biomedical solutions, such as PrEP, and the simultaneous decrease of socioeconomic safety nets and medical access, *normalizes* HIV risk for those most vulnerable" ("How to Survive" 78; "AIDS" 81). The 2014 Facebook page of the ACT UP Women's Caucus similarly identifies how racism and gender-based violence within medical narratives block access to PrEP: "PrEP's full promise can be realized only if those who need it can get it—and the topic of how women (and particularly women of color) may benefit from PrEP has been largely absent from the national public health and media discourse about this new approach to HIV." If HIV risk in particular and debility in general are *normalized* for certain people, reversing this trend prompts discussions of how everyone everywhere should have access to PrEP specifically and to medical access more broadly. In the present context of PrEP, HIV caregiving archives can continue to influence ongoing narratives about what disability is and who is unable to access this identity toward increasing body self-determination.

The tensions underlying these narratives of PrEP are further addressed by HIV activist and academic Alexander McClelland, who also identifies the history of safer sex as premised on care: "Confronting HIV back then, when it was understood as a collective responsibility, forced many queers to learn to take care of each other" (40). McClelland traces the shift from the early years of HIV where queers organized against criminalization and structural inequalities to current struggles for PrEP access, which focus instead on "demanding individual protection from people in their own communities" (43). McClelland identifies how biomedical access to PrEP and its narratives of individual responsibility for health rather than community-based practices of safer sex as care shuts down opportunities for conversations and for bonded intimacy between HIV-positive and HIV-negative partners (44; Race 17): "Fear is a rational response to the traumatic legacy of AIDS, but it's still disconnected from the realities of HIV today. . . . The grief and deaths of thousands of gay men were not taken seriously then, so how can the grief and fears of subsequent generations be taken seriously now? . . . Taking a pill might be soothing, but in the end, we can't avoid facing the past. However painful, it's part of us" (45). In "Dispatches on the Globalizations of AIDS," Ian Bradley-Perrin also identifies how PrEP "does nothing to reduce the legal burdens on poz people and does not mitigate the nondisclosure laws, thus the reduction of fear is a one-sided process. Because HIV stigma drives this product, at its very core, it *is* the product . . . the mobilization of stigma to create new markets and consumers for commodities that respond to this fear. The promise of a newly guaranteed future is marketed and consumed by our community, for our community. But it is not owned by our community" (41). In returning to early HIV community legacies of safer sex in the present, narratives of HIV caregiving can open up this space to address multigenerational trauma and fears underlying queer and trans sexuality, vulnerability, and sex (Race 14). The ongoing legacy of early HIV activism continues to offer sex education as a means of connection rather than reinforcing narratives of disability stigma or able-bodied norms.

COUNCIL OF JUDGMENT

The final section of this chapter places these safer-sex archives back into conversation with *Fledgling* to observe how disability kinships can support antiracist movements for prison abolition. HIV archives further document the labor that people of color undertook to address racism within HIV communities. As ACT UP/New York member Robert Vazquez-Pacheco recalls in his depictions of ACT UP's weekly meetings, "It was 400 white people in the room, and I would see one black man and one Mexican man over there. So we saw each other. We stood out, as my grandmother would say, like a fly in a glass of milk. We started talking to each other because we realized [we needed to] start talking about the issues of people of color" (13). Vazquez-Pacheco elaborates that the underrepresentation of people of color in these HIV communities, combined with a discomfort toward BIPOC communities and issues that affect them, contributed to access barriers for people of color both within ACT UP and in the organization's external reach. In her AIDS Activist Project oral history interview, Kim Bernard recounts her experience of being hired to work for the "all-white Coalition" of HIV organizations in the east coast of Canada. She recalls, "I thought that was a good idea that they hired somebody, but I was the only one doing it, of course. So, that presented itself with a bit of a challenge, because they sent me everywhere. I was the only one representing Black people around HIV and AIDS education work, so I kind of became what the Black community called the ambassador of HIV and AIDS in the community. [laughter] Everything that had to do with HIV/AIDS, they would call me" (5). Bernard points to the labor that falls on people of color working alone to bring issues of racism to the white group. In her oral history interview with the AIDS Activist History Project, Dionne Falconer shares her narrative of being one person in multiple roles within her organization, Toronto's Black Coalition for AIDS Prevention (Black CAP): "You know, that's how it was. I mean in community organizations you don't have the same kinds of resources, so therefore you have one person who's taking on and doing multiple things . . . and juggling multiple balls at any given point" (6). This organizational problem, as Vazquez-Pacheco recalls, affects how safer-sex information is distributed. As Ming Yuen S. Ma contends, ACT UP/New York was infused with "the larger dynamics of race and the gay community" (16) in which "community" organizing predominantly represented the interests of the white gay community, necessitating that people of color advocate for concerns and experiences overlooked by the larger group (16). Recalling the narratives of BIPOC HIV activists and their labor thus complicates the idealized narratives of HIV communities like ACT UP that are typical of many nostalgic, romanticized retellings of the early responses to HIV (Gould 57; Chen12; Juhasz and Kerr 2014; Hobson, *Lavender* 156). Exposing this fallacy of narratives that render caregiving communities as being free from outside power structures also occurs fictionally in *Fledgling*. While Shori's clan initially asserts that because vampires are "not human . . . they don't care about white or black" (168), the plot later proves not only that vampires can be outright "bigots" (292) but that some vampires' lack of alliance with Shori indicates their willingness to allow antiblack violence to continue unchecked. HIV archives thus yield narratives that frame caregiving communities not as utopias but as opportunities to address harm and violence.

Fledgling's narrative further imagines how to enact justice when antiblack racism occurs within disability communities. The caregiving provided in response to racism is ultimately represented in *Fledgling* through its extended critique of the criminal justice system. Racism, the novel suggests, cannot be addressed by the state that perpetuates it; harm could instead be mediated at the community level by drawing on the bonds of trust built among various family networks of vampires and humans via the swapping of fluids and sex. Rather than regarding prisons as a solution to violence, *Fledgling* imagines models of harm reduction that take place among kin instead of through the state. In addressing white supremacy within vampire communities, Butler's novel frames anticarceral justice as a form of care, of holding community members accountable without incarceration. In response to the antiblack violence enacted against Shori and her family, the Ina turn to their ancient practice of holding a "Council of Judgment" in order to avoid the harms of the U.S. justice system. At the Council of Judgment, a lengthy democratic Ina trial process that consumes three full days (its representation occupying seventy-one pages in the 316-page novel), some Ina refuse to protect Shori against attempts to murder her entire family line. In addition to illustrating how antiblack racism typically operates within the American legal system, the trial provides an in-depth overview of community-driven practices of anticarceral justice. Because there are "no Ina prisons" (230), punishment is imagined outside a prison system, relying instead on family power and community-based intervention. Prison abolitionists including Angela Davis and Dean Spade discuss the creation and continued function of the criminal justice system as an extension of colonial genocide and slavery into the present; Butler also takes up these questions in her slave narrative, *Kindred* (1979), using speculative fiction and time travel as a mechanism for illustrating how slavery remains central to our contemporary moment by bringing past and present together in a single narrative event. In creating this elaborate trial system, Butler's fiction imagines how justice can be achieved collaboratively as a form of care between members of affected communities rather than at the hands of the state.

Butler depicts the Ina trial against the traditional American justice system, priming the reader to become both curious about and dubious of the possibilities of achieving justice inside—and outside—of a carceral structure. Upon professing her hopes that the council's trial without imprisonment could reduce her constant fear of "another attack" (232), Shori wonders, "Could a Council of Judgment really do that? What if it couldn't?" (232). The comprehensive recounting of the council answers these queries, narrating in great detail the trial process: "We questioned each other repeatedly . . . Factual questions only. Were you told . . . ? Did you see . . . ? Did you hear . . . ? Did you scent . . . ? Did you taste . . . ? No speeches were permitted, no arguments except through questions, no interrupting each other. Preston Gordon [the council leader] could and did cut us off, though, whenever he heard us stray from these guidelines. He did this with a fairness that infuriated both Russell and me, and he paid no attention when we glared at him" (249). After many chapters of trial proceedings, sexually charged symbiont barbeque parties, and even a renegade trial-night murder, chapter 29 simply begins, "And that was that" (305). The trial ends with justice served, the well-connected Silk family of conspirators disbanded and redistributed among other families, and the universally unliked Katharine Dahlman sentenced with her noncarceral punishment: "You must, according to written law, have both your legs severed at mid-thigh" (303). Again, the vampires' status as nonhuman enables the reimagining of justice without (from before?) prisons, and Shori reminds us, "If she accepted her punishment, in a year or two, she would have legs again and be fine" (309). The significance of this punishment can also be interpreted through a crip framework which understands having one's body change to become disabled as valuable and as a different way of moving through the world rather than merely as an impairment (Murray and Bauman xv). This sentencing thus urges readers to question why disabling Katherine's body is in this instance punitive, or possibly even transformative. Potentially, the experience of living with a disability (rather than mobility changes, per se) is the lesson intended for Katherine, who understands difference as inherently impermissible. In requiring Katherine to experience temporary difference in her own body until her legs return, perhaps justice can indeed be restored. Katherine's corporeal punishment might raise further questions for readers about the transformative possibility of attaining accountability in ways that do not require incarceration. The disabling consequences Katherine receives indicate the larger sense of skepticism Butler produces about the Ina and their practices, which again cause more unease than care, a narrative process of discomfort epitomized by Shori's childlike appearance and the graphic sex she has with adults. Rather than creating a utopia, Butler instead raises questions central to the types of transformative shifts in current thinking about disability and about consent that would need to occur to create nonpunitive forms of justice. Through the fictional representation of the Council of Judgment as an alternative to prisons, *Fledgling* imagines caregiving communities not merely as enclaves away from structural oppression but as generating communally relevant responses to harm as it inevitably manifests.

As modeled by Butler's vampires, HIV archives offer ongoing narratives that reframe decriminalization and harm reduction as critical sites of care. Such narratives draw on early HIV caregiving to sustain ongoing harm reduction models with this focus on body self-determination in opposition to neoliberal models that place individual responsibility on public health. In his ACT UP Oral History interview, harm reduction activist Allan Clear recalls taking photographs of fellow ACT UP/New York member Zoe Leonard getting arrested for providing needle exchange services across the United States. These arrests were part of Leonard's two-pronged effort both to provide needles and to use her own arrests to challenge criminalization laws state by state (Leonard 29). Clear explains, "It was completely a fabricated event, and that's just another one of those brilliant things that ACT UP did. We'd been doing syringe exchange. Syringe exchange had been going on, has taken place in different parts of the city, but you just arrange this arrest. . . . We went down to Wilmington, Delaware, and got arrested down there too. . . . One of my favorite pictures is of Zoe Leonard being arrested down there" (33). (See fig. 1.4.) As Leonard depicts in her ACT UP Oral History Interview, her rage stems from witnessing "how the virus, how the disease had been made into a crisis" (180):

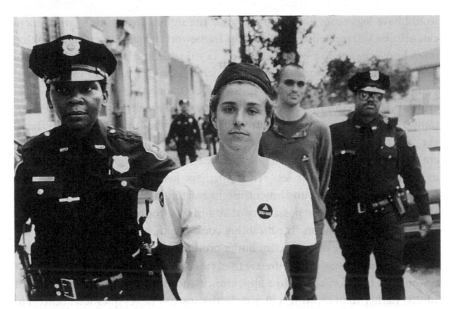

Figure 1.4. Zoe Leonard photographed by her ACT UP affinity group member Allan Clear, an image that became the cover of the *PWA Newsline*, 1991. Printed with permission from Zoe Leonard and courtesy of Allan Clear.

> It could have been over and done in two years. The first dozen people that got it or the first hundred people that got it could have been taken in and treated, and they would have died, but nobody else needed to get it and nobody else needed to die. The reason why everybody else got sick and the reason why everybody died and the reason why we have so many fucking millions of people around the world dying now is because the U.S. Government didn't want to step up and do any research, and they didn't want to do any education, and they didn't give a shit that a bunch of faggots and junkies were dying, and that it was actually a systematic genocide. It was a passive genocide. They did nothing to intervene. (21–22)

Leonard discusses the harm reduction tactics used to confront "systematic genocide" in the 1980s and early 1990s ("Surviving the AIDS Genocide" 1988). Leonard discusses her involvement in the harm reduction work of ACT UP. She explains that ACT UP was not initially working on needle exchange programs, as their initial focus was mainly on HIV and gay sex. She recalls how the inclusion of needle exchange on ACT UP's agenda was a broadening of scope that not everyone involved initially understood as important (26). Leonard's reflections on early HIV harm reduction programs also trace the relationships formed through the distribution of needles as opening up "conversations with people." Such conversations, Leonard explains, can include resource sharing: "Along with needles, you also provide condoms and answer questions that they might not be able to ask anywhere else because there was no public sex education and anything about public sex health" (27). Through decriminalizing substance use and reducing harm through community connections and health care, early HIV archives—revisited alongside *Fledgling*—provide ongoing kinship models for creating grassroots, anticarceral coalitions to address the wider access barriers brought into relief by HIV (Boucher et al. 2; Szott 182; Dodd, "Meet" 2017; Stevens and Hill; Woodland 2015).

To conclude, this chapter ultimately reads *Fledgling* to reframe caregiving toward decriminalization and prison abolition. In reimagining Butler's vampires alongside early safer-sex archives, these narratives offer ongoing community-based solutions to institutional harm. Revisiting these literary and archival texts offers ongoing queer and trans self-determination models to continue to redefine disability autonomously from the state. Taking care to decriminalize and destigmatize HIV also re-centers the goals of safer sex since its invention as a process of mutual care. This chapter combines disability narratives with speculative fiction to observe the kinships formed through negotiating the interplay of power and pleasure in the exchange of sex and of care. Building off of this chapter's investigation of early HIV archives, the following chapter returns to early trans women's print archives from the 1980s and 1990s to trace the coalitions formed through caregiving activism. Chapter 2 identifies the absence of trans women's narratives in HIV archives to re-center the administrative, emotional, and caregiving labor undertaken by trans women's communities responding to disability. In these chapters and throughout this book, narratives of the vulnerabilities of interdependence of HIV caregiving reframe disability not as a site of shame but as inspiring ongoing anticapitalist formations for supporting chosen family and body self-determination.

CHAPTER 2

Caregiving Collations and "Gender Trash from Hell"

TRANS WOMEN'S HIV ARCHIVES

In a 1991 issue of the *New York Times*, ACT UP/New York ran a full-page advertisement that reads in bold font, "Women Don't Get AIDS / They Just Die from It." This ad confronts the original Centers for Disease Control (CDC) definitions of AIDS as primarily concerning men. Symptoms of AIDS not experienced by men, such as pulmonary tuberculosis, were omitted from original CDC definitions, creating a medical climate wherein women living with HIV were not being diagnosed, researched, or granted access to care (Denenberg, "Unique Aspects" 32–33; Christensen, "How do Women Live" 5). Such gendered definitions of HIV render women as vectors and victims rather than as subjects with tangible access needs (Charlesworth 2; McCarthy and Kirschenbaum 34; Hogan 3). Women are criminalized as infectious and rendered by medical literature as existing sexually for procreation or for the pleasure of others rather than as agents in seeking pleasure and care (Charlesworth 5–7; Gilman 2; P. Levine 293; Maher et al. 5). Faced with this medical gendering of illness, queer women began conducting their own research on HIV and publishing their findings in community periodicals including the "In Our Own Hands" column of *Outweek* magazine. HIV activists, including the ACT UP's Women's Caucus that placed the full-page ad in the *Times*, responded to medical neglect by making media, creating support groups, filing prisoner-led lawsuits, and launching direct action campaigns to change CDC definitions that excluded women from access to treatment, clinical studies, education, and health insurance (Denenberg, "Treatment" 74; Christensen, "How do Women Live" 5; Denenberg, "What the Numbers Mean" 3; Cheairs et al. 12). These caregiving activists made clear that due to the CDC's AIDS definitions, women were being misdiagnosed and diagnosed late and were consequently dying faster than men (Pearl 4). While such activist campaigns were successful in expanding the CDC's definitions to better include cisgender women, the lack of inclusion of trans women within these queer HIV movements creates an ongoing gendering of HIV that continues to block access to care.

UNBURYING

This chapter revisits early HIV archives to address this exclusion of trans women from queer HIV organizing and archiving practices. Extending from chapter 1's analysis of vampire fiction and safer-sex histories as narratives of caregiving, unburying these archives connects early HIV narratives to ongoing models of disability kinship. This chapter starts with a return to trans women's archival newsletters from the 1980s and early 1990s to unearth caregiving narratives of coalition building in response to HIV. I next analyze the HIV caregiving communities documented within contemporary narratives commemorating the work of trans performing artists and long-term survivors of HIV. I connect these legacies to the ongoing activism and archives of trans HIV organizing, and to the production of 1990s zines and video that address rifts between trans women's and gay men's communities. Reading these varied texts together broadens definitions of caregiving to include the sharing of information for sexual and gender self-determination into the present. Trans women's HIV archives contain narratives of the care-based, administrative, and emotional work of coalition building, gendered labor that is often undervalued in spite of its impact of preventing isolation. A return to archival trans women's self-documentations address gender-based violence through kinship formations in response to disability. Trans women's care work not only brings individuals together but also forms connections between separate communities needing to access similar medical and support services. Disability becomes impetus for building gay and trans community alliances toward de-pathologizing bodies that disrupt medical as well as gender norms. Rather than reductively framing illness as a problem to be cured, these archives offer narratives of disability as opportunity to expand trans leadership and institutional access while also addressing broken relationships between gay men's and trans women's communities. These HIV narratives do not reveal easy alliances between gay and trans organizing but rather narrate the potential of ongoing caregiving coalitions to reconceive body norms in response to disability.

Unearthing these trans women's caregiving narratives raises concerns of memory and preservation, as HIV archiving practices call attention to which histories are now locatable versus which narratives remain unfindable or erased. Scholars including Ann Cvetkovich have demonstrated the historical impact of the New York Public Library's (NYPL) HIV archives as well as the community-building prospects of these collections (Cvetkovich 246). Queer scholarship also connects these collections to Brooklyn's Lesbian Herstory Archives, which feature an extensive women and HIV history in periodicals, posters, and other original documents. Such collections include the Lesbian AIDS Project (LAP)'s original 1990s poster campaign, in which a 1950s-style illustrated cross-racial dyke couple shares an intimate conversation relayed through a pair of speech bubbles: "I don't know any lesbians with AIDS / Now you do" (see fig. 2.1.). In spite of the impressive array of materials preserved in these holdings, the activist histories of trans women within these collections remain absent. This erasure reflects larger processes of transmisogyny, whereby cisgender lesbians have excluded trans women from their organizing and spaces (M. Page 2012; Serano 5). Trans historian Susan Stryker identifies trans women's pivotal contributions to HIV activism and community resistance (*Transgender History* 132). She outlines how trans women's work within HIV activist movements not only was essential in fighting medical injustices but also contributed significantly to women's cultural histories and the expansion of gender expressions within queer organizing (134). Stryker identifies HIV activism as enabling the birth of *queer* as an "unabashedly progay, nonseparatist, antiassimilationist alliance politics to combat AIDS" (Stryker, *Transgender History* 134; Gould 66). She traces how this shift in gay, lesbian, and bisexual internal politics allowed trans politics to return into the community's dialogue, uniting sexual and gender movements that had been heavily fractured since the unifying political moments surrounding Stonewall (Stryker, *Transgender History* 134; Gould 5; Cvetkovich 159; Hallas 26; Leonard 12; Muñoz 47; Rollerena 41, 55). Stryker additionally points to the role of HIV in "revitalizing the transgender movement" (132) by providing outreach, support, services, funding, education, job opportunities, and social venues to trans communities that were already facing barriers to resource access (132). Revisiting trans women's early writing about HIV thus offers ongoing narratives of caregiving in response to disability as generating kinships for gender self-determination into the present.

Early HIV archives also document the medical narratives through which HIV was initially gendered. Trans women were erased within both the mainstream medical literature and within narratives of HIV activism. These exclusionary narratives of women and HIV can thus be addressed by re-centering archival histories of trans women's HIV caregiving as a critical component of HIV storytelling. The impact of narratives in defining what HIV is and whom HIV affects shapes current cultural understandings of disability access. Revisiting the early HIV archives thus offers further narrative opportunities to challenge this ongoing exclusion of trans women that originates with the initial gendering of HIV. Addressing these issues of medical exclusion in a contemporary moment, Cecilia Chung, a San Francisco–based long-term survivor, discusses her activism in confronting this gender-based violence. In a 2013 interview for *The Body*, Chung

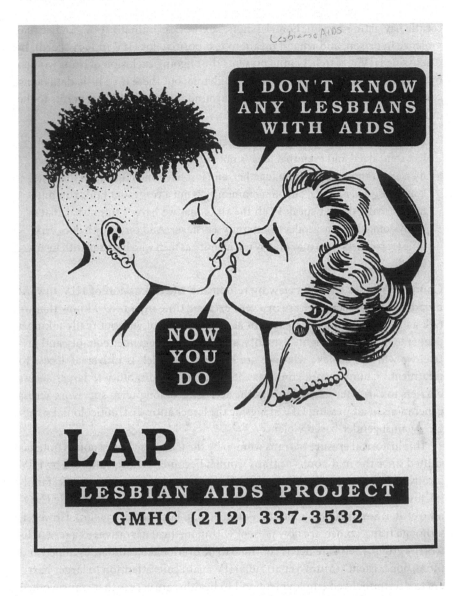

Figure 2.1. Lesbian AIDS Project (LAP) poster, filed under "Lesbians & AIDS," at the Lesbian Herstory Archives, Brooklyn, NY. Courtesy of Lesbian Herstory Archives.

recalls navigating racism, homelessness, sex work criminalization, and sexual violence in prison, and what it meant to test positive for HIV in 1993 (Ford). In discussing HIV research, Chung presents the ongoing exclusion of trans women by the CDC: "We have 30 years in the epidemic, but there is so little data being collected in the transgender community around the world." Chung points to the current limits of medical data collection:

> It wasn't until recently that the US Centers for Disease Control decided to collect some data, and even that data is not segregated. They lump transgender men and transgender women together, and just have one single item that lists it as *transgender people*, but our community is not a very monolithic community. It really doesn't speak to all the risks that we have. I think that that's really doing the transgender community a disfavor. And certainly it does very little for partners, who may or may not identify as men who have sex with men. (Ford)

Chung concludes her interview by refocusing the discussion of HIV toward broader access issues: "We are in a very exciting time right now. I know that we talk a lot about treatment, treatment as prevention, but without really taking a deeper look at human rights, equality, and really about gender equality and justice, we will not achieve what we are looking at, which is universal access to treatment." Chung's work connects the gendering of disability to larger access barriers to care. Her writing brings the activisms of long-term survivors across generations in addressing HIV alongside the larger antiracist, anticolonial struggles against gender-based violence.

This historical erasure of trans women by the CDC, as Chung points out, has shifted since the mid-2000s as trans women become visible as affected by HIV locally and transnationally because of wider systemic barriers to economic, familial, and health-care access (Munro et al. 708; Turner et al. 2; Pacifico de Carvalho et al. 1; Sevelius et al. 1060–61; Poteat et al. 1; Jaspal et al. 239–40). However, although trans women are now present within medical narratives as a research-worthy group, their care needs continue to be overlooked, "underdeveloped and often, nonexistent" (Munro et al. 718). HIV again calls attention to larger barriers to decriminalized employment and to health-care access that trans women of color face, and to the harms of misgendering trans women through the construction of HIV research classifications like that of "Men Who Have Sex with Men (MSM)": "As the history of HIV prevention and treatment research has demonstrated, trans women have been left behind . . . and they have higher rates of HIV than any group as well as higher rates of morbidity and mortality. . . . To date, PrEP [pre-exposure prophylaxis] research has repeated this pattern" (Sevelius et al. 1063). "It cannot be overstated," argue Poteat et al., "that transgender women are not MSM and should not be subsumed in a category that erases their identity. Likewise, transgender MSM should be visible within the data about

MSM" (3). Retuning to trans women's early HIV caregiving narratives thus resists contemporary narratives that frame HIV care for trans women as a recently emerging phenomenon newly identified by medical researchers working from outside of trans women's communities. Early HIV narratives, on the contrary, position the contemporary movements to address gender-based access barriers as part of the ongoing caregiving labor of trans women who have been working all along, even when erased by the CDC, to address HIV toward leveraging broader coalitions for trans body self-determination.

AREAS WHERE OUR INTERESTS OVERLAP

In this section, I undertake a return to trans women's newsletters that address coalition building and disability in relation to HIV. Revisiting these archives through the lens of caregiving thus connects contemporary movements for trans access to early narratives of gender and HIV. In revisiting archives of trans women's HIV coalitions that formed in the past, these narrative models continue to shape disability kinships in the present. Understanding HIV as opportunity for coalition building reframes disability as an ongoing opportunity to challenge gender norms. These archives contain narratives about care that counter the isolation and medical shame faced by gender nonconforming bodies. In *Histories of the Transgender Child*, Jules Gill-Peterson revisits the archive to demonstrate how trans children shaped the biomedical discourse about gender in order to assert their own medical desires and body self-determinations: although these children understood their bodies as trans without yet encountering biomedicine, "medicine was significantly challenged by its encounters with them" (Gill-Peterson, *Histories* 95). Following Gill-Peterson's work, a return to the archive demonstrates how medical narratives about HIV are shaped by trans narratives of body self-determination. In connecting trans women's specific HIV organizing to that of other queer communities, the range of bodies supported by disability activism can continue to rescript biomedical narratives that shame gender and sexual self-expression.

HIV narratives for body self-determination can be found within a series of trans women's archival newsletters from the 1980s and 1990s, periodical collections that are now housed in the University of Victoria's Transgender Archives and at the ArQuives. These HIV narratives address community divides but also imagine coalitions in response to accessing care. HIV is framed not as creating easy alliances between trans and gay communities but as opening up conversations about connections between the medicalization of gender and the pathologization of queer sexuality through discussions of disability. In reframing biomedical stigma as motivating cross-community coalitions, these archives inspire ongoing caregiving kinships premised on increasing disability access. One such narrative of HIV as a point of community cohesion can be found within *Girl Talk*, a newsletter published by the Powder Puffs of California, an organization "serving the California gender community since 1987" (1). *Girl Talk's* twelfth volume from 1997 devotes a feature article to the corresponding struggles between HIV activism and trans activism. *Girl Talk* columnist Melanie Yarborough maps points of commonality between gay and trans organizing (2). She draws parallels in relation to medical access: "The gay community must deal with the slow and frustrating medical bureaucracy on issues of AIDS research. The Transsexual community must deal with the slow and frustrating medical bureaucracy on issues of hormone therapy and sexual reassignment surgery" (2). Yarborough's article validates the mutual distrust between these two communities while noting points of overlap for coalition building. She closes her analysis by proposing, "It's time we put aside our differences, started to dialogue, and worked together" (2). HIV narratives offer this model for identifying points of unification between experiences of sexuality- and gender-based access barriers to care. This early HIV narrative opens discussions of how communities with unequal access to resources might work through distrust or find points of common organizing. *Girl Talk* narrates care not as dispensed solely from "slow and frustrating medical bureaucracy" but as community driven and supported. These newsletters center community audiences through HIV narratives advocating for the self-directed care necessitated by state neglect.

HIV narratives thus play a critical role in the process of identifying the gender and sexual dimensions of disability access. These archives contain narrative histories of taking back care from the hands of the state. Another example of this process of reframing disability as a point of gay and trans community cohesion can be found in Houston's trans women's periodical, *The Gulf Coast Transgender Community: An Outreach Organization (GCTC)* (see fig. 2.2.). In an issue from 1995, HIV is again depicted via narratives identifying the institutional neglect in failing to provide care for people living with HIV. This newsletter addresses its trans readership by conjuring a collective sense of queer accountability, "since the so called 'straight' community has chosen to abrogate their responsibility to the people who are afflicted with this disease" (March 1995, vol. 8, no. 3, p. 6). Whereas discussions of being "afflicted" by HIV certainly cast disability as an undesirable experience, the column shifts from narratives of affliction toward reframing disability as that which motivates unification between gay and trans communities. In discussing rifts between gay/lesbian and trans organizing, the editors ask,

Why is it so hard for the gender community to work with the gay and lesbian community? I realize most of us are not gay. (Truth be known, there are probably a whole lot more people who are bi-sexual than care to own up to it, but that is another story for another time.) Sexual orientation is what defines the gay and lesbian community. Gender identity or preference is what defines

EVENTS CALENDAR

Date	Location	Event	Program
9 May	Linda's Beach House	Meeting Parrrty	Beach Part
12 May	Feagans Restaurant	Law & Program Committees	Help Plan
19 May	Feagans Restaurant	Board Meeting	
26 May	Feagans Restaurant	Law & Program Committees	Help Plan
2 Jun	Feagans Restaurant	Law & Program Committees	Help Plan
13 Jun	TBA	Meeting	Religious Guilt
11 Jul	TBA	Meeting	Significant Others
08 Aug	TBA	Meeting	Fashion Show

Business cards with this logo, the name, address and phone number will be printed up and made available to members.

FANTASY ADVENTURE WEEKEND

The officers and board discussed the idea of resurrecting the Fantasy Adventure weekend. It was agreed it would be impossible at this late date to even consider putting one on this year. With the IFGE convention and International Law Conference in August, we leave all we can handle this year. As far as 1993, it was decided to leave this in the officers and board that will be

elected in November of 1992. They would have the benefit of a full year to plan and coordinate it, if they chose to do so. They would also be able to judge whether they could handle the FAW as well as the Second Law Conference which is tentatively planned for August of 1993.

NOMINATIONS AND ELECTIONS

Even though the GCTC elections are still six months away, it is not too early to begin thinking about whether you may want to run for one of the officer or board positions. The President and Vice President will not have an incumbent running. The Editor of the Newsletter or Secretary/Treas-

Unfortunately, due to the dates of the convention (April 6th thru 13th), I was able to attend a more limited number of events than I would have

legislator just does not have time to personally talk to everyone that might wish to lobby them for their own personal agenda. A fashion show,

PRESIDENT'S PERSPECTIVE

Whew!!! The IFGE convention is over. From all indications it was highly successful. I want to acknowledge some of the people who worked to make it happen so smoothly as it did. A committee was formed back in September to handle the local aspects of the event. Heading it up were Sheri Lee Summers and Joan Bray. They were assisted by myself, Vivian McKenzie, Cynthia Davis, Linda & Peggy Carter, Taylor & Rebecca McGowan, and yours truly from G.C.T.C. They served on such diverse subcommittees as Events, Contacts, Media Relations, Keynote Speakers & Decorations among others. Additional workers on the subcommittees included Jamie Ward, Phyllis Frye, Rene Fenner, Cynthia Lee, Karen Thomas, JoAnne Roberts, Tammy Huemme, Amber Daugherty, Regina Corder and Ruby Gonzales. All in all, a very commendable contribution of time and effort by the members of G.C.T.C.

Meeting Date : 9 May
Meeting Place : Linda's Beach House
Galveston
Noon Till...
See Map

Board Meeting :
19 May   7:00 PM
Feagans Restaurant
404 Shepard & Feagan

Law Confrence Committees 7:00
Program Committee Meetings 8:00
12 May - 26 May - 2 June
Feagans Restaurant
404 Shepard & Feagan

liked to. But I was able to attend the seminar that was open to the public on Tuesday night which discussed the various aspects of transgenderism. It was well attended and there were several local counselors and psychologists there. Needless to say, they came away with a much expanded understanding of what's been talked about. Thursday's lunch featured State Representative Debra Danburg, who spoke on how to approach members of the state legislature to obtain favorable (or still adverse) laws. The real secret is to approach the staff people, as the

in which several of our members were models, was presented also.

I could not attend the social at Missouri Street Station on Thursday or the charitable fundraiser on Friday. I understand that both were great fun, with the benefit raising $1,780. for the AIDS foundation of Houston, the local charity of our efforts. Congratulations are certainly in order for all involved, but especially for Joan, who lined up both events.

Figure 2.2.   The Gulf Coast Transgender Community (GCTC) newsletter informs readers of an upcoming meeting parrrty (1991). *The GCTC Transmission Line: Newsletter of the Gulf Coast Transgender Community,* January 1991, courtesy of University of Victoria Libraries, Transgender Archives, Call # HQ77.9 T7866.

the gender community. There are a whole bunch of areas where our interests overlap. We should be concentrating on those points we have in common rather than our differences. (6)

In identifying "those points we have in common," these newsletters represent HIV as motivation to link gender-based and sexual oppression via caregiving activism. Disability is thus framed not simply as an individual embodiment but as a collective opportunity to intervene in neglect by the state. This model of body self-determination in opposition to state systems can continue to support ongoing queer and trans disability movements today.

In identifying these medical points of overlap between gay and trans access needs, these newsletters addressing HIV frame disability as motivation for extending community. This mode of narrating HIV as opportunity for bridging gay and trans movements appears across a range of other trans women's periodicals from the 1980s and 1990s. Discussions of disability as a point of trans community cohesion appear in *Our Sorority*, a trans women's newsletter edited by Betty Ann Lind that first appeared in 1980 and ran for over a decade. Issue 21 from January 1990 features an excerpt from a progress report assessing the access needs of trans women's communities in a range of areas including funding, service provision, and community support forums. In addressing the area of "helping professionals," this newsletter again frames HIV as a point of overlap with gay communities. The article identifies how "the AIDS epidemic has been particularly destructive of the drag community and its bridging into the straight community via bisexualism, most often marked by crossdressing behavior" ("Future" 6). The author traces how stigma and blame are placed upon trans and gender nonconforming women for "spreading" the virus to the "straight community" who "naively believes that it is immune" (16). Trans identities, as a result, become the site of "fear of AIDS" (7) via narratives that conflate gender transgression with illness. Such links between gender-based and sexual discrimination motivate ongoing gay and trans community unification in response to disability stigma.

These newsletters directly address trans medicalization as it creates disability stigma. Through a comparison between trans women's access barriers and those of gay men, this *Our Sorority* article points to a further contrast between gender and sexual oppression. The author identifies "the psychiatric *normalization* of being gay" as "a battle won" (6) that allows gay men to occupy a public rather than closeted existence. The authors identify narratives linking trans identity with illness stigma as a locus of trans shame. These newsletters thereby suggest that in order to counter the conflation of trans-ness with disability, communities must expose this narrative process. A later issue of *Our Sorority* from 1991 features an excerpt of newsletter editor Lind's public address on receiving the Virginia Prince Award for trans leadership. Her acceptance speech touches on issues ranging from coalition building with gay communities and "among our 'drag' sisters" ("Dever" 16), to economic development and access to legal defense. Lind asserts, "Whether we are transsexuals, or any other form of CD [cross-dresser] we should never claim that as a 'disability,' no matter how economically tempting that may be. Because it classifies us as 'sick.' These CD's are playing into the hands of our enemies by proving to the world that we lack the ability to help ourselves. The distance between being 'sick' and being 'deviant' is less than the thickness of a human hair" (17). Lind's imperative here can be further complicated through Douglas Baynton's theoretical work on disability: Baynton conducts an analysis of groups who are classified as disabled that organize to remove themselves from this category in order to mark their differences not as pathological but as the result of prejudice and negative stereotyping (38). Such desires to remove the stigmatized label of disability, however, risk rendering those who are disabled as undeserving of rights granted to those classified as able-bodied (Baynton 38). Bringing these narratives of trans-ness and disability into the present can sustain an ongoing coalition between trans and disability organizing. For instance, AJ Withers's contemporary crip theory critiques the medical model that regards trans-ness *as* disability for overlooking the ways in which many trans people (beyond their medical classification as trans) are also disabled. As Withers attests, it is not until queer and trans communities focus on increasing access for those trans and queer community members who are also disabled that disability can be reclaimed as a collective site of power rather than as a site of shame (*Disability* 100).

In returning to the early HIV archive to bring these two categories of identity together, these trans caregiving legacies can continue to challenge medical narratives that pathologize bodies marked as different. Tracing the narrative medicalization of trans identities offers an opportunity not only to destigmatize gender nonconforming bodies but also to reframe narratives of disability shame. In *Sex Change, Social Change*, Viviane Namaste outlines how trans women navigate gender-based violence alongside experiences of disability, as disability intersects with poverty and with the criminalization of employment like sex work (134). Namaste discusses the disabling effects of the lack of institutional support for a broad range of trans women's access needs including but not limited to health care (134). Namaste also traces the process by which access to gender-confirming health care in Ontario required legally claiming trans-ness as a disability (172), depicting how understandings of being trans as a disability are connected to health insurance legislation as access to care. Taking up these issues in an American context, Eli Clare discusses this classification of trans-ness as a disability in a system where health insurance is private and thus a disability listing may lead not to free health care but to increased gatekeeping. Clare traces the process by which narratives of cure for the "problem" of being trans were created by the medical gatekeeping processes that originally framed trans-ness as a "defect" (*Brilliant* 177): "Until the early 1990s, when trans communities began finding strong, collective voices, medical providers' explicit goal for gender transition was to create normal heterosexual men and women who never again identified as trans, gender-nonconforming, gay, lesbian, or bi. In other words, the framing of transness as defect, an abnormality to be corrected, didn't start with trans people but with the medical-industrial complex" (178). Clare addresses the *Diagnostic and Statistical Manual*'s (DSM) initial creation of trans-ness as pathological and as subject to medical gatekeeping through diagnostic categories like "gender identity disorder" (gid) and the more recent "gender dysphoria" (gd) (179). Clare writes, "Many trans activists pose fundamental challenges to gid and gd. We want to know why these diagnoses live in the dsm. We object to the ways in which the medical-industrial complex defines our genders as disordered. We resist the pathology foisted on us. And yet I want us to reach farther: to imagine dismantling the dsm itself, discarding the concepts of disorder and defect, and developing other means of accessing medical technology beyond white Western diagnosis. Yes, I am suggesting a rebellion" (142). Clare's call for "rebellion" can be read in connection with Baynton's directive to understand disability classifications not as opportunities to remove oneself from such a classification but rather as means to create improved care for all those who are disabled by medical gatekeeping, by capitalism, and by cultural definitions of health. Returning to early HIV archives can further incite such a rebellion to find power in bodily differences that come not only through gender and sexual resistance but through the reframing of disability via the ongoing history of HIV. Quoting Alexandre Baril, Clare argues, "The problem with framing transness as a defect resides, I believe, not in the concept of transness as disability, but in such individualist, ableist, pathologising views of disabilities" (178). As Clare illustrates, the stigma associated with disability and the prevalence of "promises of cure" (8) prevent all those marked as disabled from building coalitions by claiming the label without shame. As Gould identifies, collective anger transforms feelings of internalized anti-queer violence ("shame on us") into feelings of entitlement to resource access ("shame on you") (46). As Taryn Jordan discusses in her research on black rage, collective responses to violence against black bodies can open up the potential to "provide useful ruptures that bring people together" (12). This model demonstrates that anger as an affective force is not simply reactive but also generative to movements including Black Lives Matter. A return to trans HIV archives thus offers narrative models of ongoing antiracist, anticapitalist, and disability coalitions to continue to create kinships in response to body norms.

Because I belong to a generation that could not participate in HIV caregiving during this period, I read these newsletters as an opportunity for my own and for younger generations to learn from these discussions of illness and loss.

In forming trans support groups and coalitions in response to disability and death, these narratives further expand definitions of care. Trans narratives of disability reframe the act of providing support—for community members facing the loss of multiple friends and lovers to AIDS and other forms of structural violence—as a critical exchange of care. Caregiving is not represented as an easy process but as a site of vulnerability, pain, and grief. The representations of HIV caregiving in these newsletters could transmit these narratives across generations; these publications might also inspire ongoing community formations to support people who—including those in older generations who lost friends and lovers to AIDS—are experiencing mourning. These newsletters discuss the challenges of living with illness while also providing representations of dying and grief. Such narratives both recognize the pain of illness and loss and acknowledge the forms of unification that coalesce in response to HIV. In her *GCTC's* column "Jet Trails" from 1995, columnist Jackie Evelyn Thorne connects trans and gay communities through the act of mourning. She discusses "the number of female impersonators (mostly from the gay community, but also transgendered) who have passed away from AIDS" (6). Documenting how her experience and years in the trans community allow her to understand the duration and scope of this loss, she muses, "Let's face it, we're both older than dirt!" (6), pushing conversations between senior members of the community regarding sexual risk. In a later article, from 1996, Thorne again discusses performance as a venue "that had allowed [her] to be who [she] really was" (6), and that also became a fundraising strategy for HIV access and care. Thorne's sentiments echo those in an earlier issue of *En Femme Magazine*, a trans women's newsletter from 1988. *En Femme* documents the involvement of trans women in creating fundraising events for HIV caregiving that doubled as drag shows for trans community building and support (38) (see fig. 2.3.). Thorne cautions that though fundraising and support work addressing HIV is essential, it should not erase the need to respond to other illnesses including cancer (6). In framing disability as incentive for community cohesion, these newsletters again provide narratives that move beyond stigma and shame and toward understanding disability as generating community formation in response to death and loss.

As in the safer-sex archives of chapter 1, the trans narratives within these newsletters also expand definitions of caregiving to include access to sexual health education. Chapter 1 returns to HIV archives to locate the invention of safer sex as a practice not of public health shaming but rather one premised on care; through narratives published for purposes of community cohesion, trans women's newsletters also evidence the caregiving labor of confronting HIV stigma as connected to wider access barriers. These newsletters discuss the need for community gatherings in which to talk openly about sexuality and sex. In creating these spaces, trans community members care for one another through

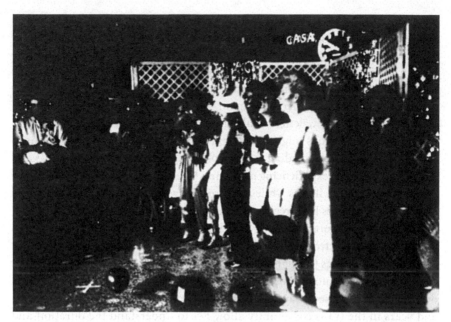

Figure 2.3. *The Cast Takes Their Final Bow*, a photo concluding *En Femme*'s eight-page documentation of the AIDS benefit (1988). *En Femme* magazine, May/Jun 1988, courtesy of University of Victoria Libraries, Transgender Archives, Call # HQ77.9 E45.

the exchange of information. This process is documented within the text of the newsletters themselves. Urging readers to be "active in the cause of AIDS eradication" (8), the *GCTC* presents sex-positive conversations about HIV as a tool for community building. In a March 1996 review of a workshop given to *GCTC* members by the AIDS Foundation, Vivian McKenzie explains the importance of providing accessible, community-based venues for HIV education. McKenzie muses on the workshop's intermission wherein the women took a break from discussing sex acts and transmission routes to eat. She shares, "Kenny used several props for the workshop, and his very life-like phallus made for a rather bizarre centerpiece standing proudly amongst the flowers and candles" (1). McKenzie recounts the workshop's ending, complete with "lots of party favors which reminded [her] of the joke about a note on a men's room condom machine which said 'Don't buy this gum. It tastes like rubber'" (1). While the workshop does sex education in real time, the newsletter provides an ongoing space to continue these sex-positive HIV discussions within trans women's communities. The newsletter's narrative further involves trans community members in HIV conversations even if they missed the in-person event. As contemporary readers of these archival documents, we are included in these trans community narratives across time and space. Revisiting these early HIV archives thus inspires ongoing queer and trans community formations in response to disability.

CAREGIVING FAILS

In moving from an investigation of archival newsletters to contemporary media memorializing trans women's HIV activism, this next section reads works commemorating long-term survivors of HIV. Examining the narratives of caregiving preserved within HIV archives again raises questions of which narratives of gendered labor are not housed within these material histories. Whereas the AIDS Activist History Project and the NYPL's archives preserve cis women's interventions into gendered medical narratives, the work of trans women in response to HIV remains absent from these collections. Extending on the narratives preserved in trans women's print newsletters, revisiting early HIV archives reanimates the caregiving activisms about gender that are archivally missing. This return to the caregiving work of trans women within archives of HIV activism is the subject of *Duets: Che Gossett & Alice O'Malley in Conversation on Chloe Dzubilo*. This Visual AIDS publication commemorates the legacy of visual artist, trans advocate, punk performer, and HIV long-term survivor and activist Chloe Dzubilo, who died in 2011. Writer and archivist Che Gossett and portrait photographer Alice O'Malley link trans women's activism to ongoing issues of HIV stigma. They attest, "Chloe saw the struggle against transphobia as part of a larger struggle against violent 'systems.' . . . In thinking about the legacy and struggle by trans AIDS activists, how can trans communities and gender self-determination be more centered around HIV prevention and treatment services and in AIDS activism?" (43–44). In memorializing the work of Dzubilo, Gossett and O'Malley frame trans activism and HIV activism as together advocating mutually for gender and sexual self-determination. They argue, "We can take inspiration from Chloe's liberation of language and think about how to talk about AIDS prevention and health care in ways that don't reinforce shame and sex negativity. How often have I gone to the doctor's office and heard the doctor using risk rhetoric, which can reinforce queer shame? Chloe helps us to think in more liberatory ways" (33). Gossett and O'Malley approach trans women's archives as inspiring the ongoing sexual and gender liberation work of HIV activism from the past and into contemporary modes of reimagining disability, chosen family, and health-care access. *Duets* also presents an interview with Dzubilo in which she discusses her role in building community through health-care activism: "I was also working on the frontlines of the trans movement in the nineties. I would listen to trans women talk about their horrible experiences. Many didn't want to even go to doctors or had been treated like freaks" (12). Dzubilo also connects her experience of disability to her creative practice. She shares, "I want to make my work larger. The work I've done was mostly created from being in bed. I have terrible neuropathy and live with a lot of chronic bone pain. The works are mostly small, because I work where I live, in a studio apartment" (13). Re-centering Dzubilo's once-domestic work as part of a public HIV archive creates opportunities for bringing trans women's caregiving activisms into a lineage of ongoing disability movements.

Returning now to Dzubilo's art and narratives of trans medical resistance bridges HIV caregiving archives with ongoing models of disability kinship by expanding the range of narratives that exist within the HIV archive itself. As Kate Eichhorn explains, "what makes the archive a potential site of resistance is arguably not simply its mandate or its location but rather how it is deployed in the present" (160). Unburying archives like Dzubilo's, argues Eichhorn, allows for a reconstruction of not "the worlds these collections claim to represent, but rather the worlds they invite us to imagine and even realize" (160). Gossett and O'Malley discuss Dzubilo's punk band Transisters as emblematizing narratives of HIV as a collective site of power rather than as site of shame:

> ALICE: One of her songs was called Kaposi Coverstick.
> CHE: Meaning using makeup to cover Kaposi's sarcoma lesions?
> ALICE: Yes! She was public about her HIV status onstage, which was radical. (33)

These memories of Dzubilo also situate her art and activist work alongside her role as a community caregiver and as a recipient of community care. In his foreword to *Duets*, New York–based writer JP Borum emphasizes, "Chloe's art isn't about isolated genius. It's about being part of a community" (16). Gossett asserts that Dzubilo was "failed by systems of care," emphasizing the ongoing need to increase medical access and community supports for long-term survivors of HIV. Regarding health-care access for trans women, Dzubilo also depicts her own experience of medical violence and abuse from health-care practitioners. She connects surviving these experiences to the process of creating art: "I also used to draw pictures of things that were happening that would really upset me. Like dealing with being trans in the healthcare machine. Even in the hospital, though, there would be creative stuff going on" (12). The hospital can become the locus both of trauma and of transmitting experience toward the formation of communities of care. Disability communities serve as supports for navigating the "healthcare machine." Rather than leave these texts in the past, this archive can be reanimated toward "being in time differently" (x), not "to escape the present but rather as an attempt to regain agency in an era when the ability to collectively imagine and enact other ways of being in the world has become deeply eroded" (Eichhorn 9). Eichhorn imagines time as being "dispersed across different eras and generations" (x). I hope, as a member of a younger generation learning from Dzubilo's work, to extend on her art and activism to also consider what happens when the amount of care available is insufficient.

The trans HIV archive thus also remains important precisely because it offers ongoing narrative strategies for addressing caregiving's limitations. Michelle Lawler's 2009 documentary film, *Forever's Gonna Start Tonight*, represents disability narratives that center the isolating experiences of daily stigma and pain.

Revisiting Dzubilo's narratives of caregiving failures alongside this documentary considers what archival narratives can do to help reconcile models of queer and trans disability kinship with these very real limitations of care. Lawler's documentary commemorates the life and work of Vicki Marlane, who was seventy-one years old at the time of the film's shooting (Marlane died in 2011 at the age of seventy-seven). In the film, Marlane recollects growing up as a trans girl in the 1930s and 1940s, being criminalized and imprisoned under anti-trans and anti–sex work laws, working in the carnival circuit in freak shows, starring in drag performances in strip clubs, and living with disabilities including HIV. The archival turn Eichhorn investigates is again a central tactic within Lawler's film. Lawler presents layered footage of Marlane's current drag performances with findings from the archive. The archival photographs presented are annotated by voiceovers from Marlane's interviews for the film, creating a familiar documentary style of autobiographical narration. In one trans archival photograph, a group of friends sit around a dinner table in 1974. Marlane is able to recall everyone in the group from left to right (save for, she says, "the two next to me, I really don't know who they were"). As the camera zooms in on the photo and pans from one side to the other, Marlane recalls each name, explaining that now everyone is gone. Marlane then itemizes the cause of all her friends' deaths: diabetes, heart attacks, AIDS. The camera then returns to the source of the voice, Marlane posed casually in a t-shirt and a ponytail, interviewing on her sofa in a sunny living room: "I'm surprised I'm still here." The narrative presents a discrepancy between the carefree glamour of the archival material and Marlane's ongoing, day-to-day experience of disability: "Some days I feel fine, and other days I can't get out of bed." The camera captures Marlane's seemingly immortal trans performances but then points to the ways Marlane's living body experiences long-term chronic pain, a state that remains undetectable visually by the camera and is conveyed only through Marlane's accompanying commentary. While the camera documents the dance feats performed by Marlane's aging body, Marlane's voiceover explains that she needs to sit down between acts because of the sciatic nerve in her leg: "I can't hardly walk more than a block or so at a time; it starts killing me." Marlane lists her body's limits, then adds, "Other than that, other than falling apart . . . my whole body's falling apart now." The video and audio together create a mix of resilience and pain that characterizes Marlane's performances themselves. Marlane then performs to the opening track of the film, its titular song, explaining, "That's why I like that song, it's my life story." The film traces this life story in a linear progression from childhood to the present, including Marlane's experience of being diagnosed with HIV following a suicide attempt in the 1980s. Marlane explains how drag performance and drag community saved her life: "If I didn't do it I'd be dead. I'd be sitting here day and night. At least now I've got my Fridays and Saturdays to look forward to." This discrepancy between the nostalgia of the past and the resilience of the present becomes a narrative strategy of the archival film in showing how care can simultaneously support and fail to break isolation. In grappling with the pleasure and the pain that come from queer and trans disability kinships, the film animates the archive to represent how these communities are unable to eliminate the daily challenges of navigating systems and illness: the archive opens up a space to continue to imagine the kind of networks needed to better care for those experiencing gender-based violence alongside long-term, chronic pain. Returning to trans women's HIV archives including those of long-term survivors, Dzubilo and Marlane envision a future of collective care in opposition to neoliberal ideas of medical cure and individual responsibility for health. Such connections are important because, as Dzubilo and Marlane's autobiographical narratives indicate, navigating disability with feelings of loneliness can increase suffering. These archives re-center the process of coalition building, caregiving, and mutual aid as strategies that increase disability access in spite of institutional failures to provide care. These archives demonstrate how isolation can increasingly be broken through narratives that understand disability not as a site of individual responsibility or shame but as opportunity for kinship. Such kinships are not isolated to these early responses to HIV but continue today.

For People Being Ignored by the System

Building from this investigation of trans newsletters, interviews, and documentary film, this section now returns again to the early archive of HIV. Recentering trans women's caregiving and administrative labor within early responses to HIV connects caregiving activism in the past to ongoing queer and trans movements for body self-determination. Finding such records requires searching outside of the NYPL and HIV collections that exclude trans women's work from their HIV archiving practices. Housed within San Francisco's GLBT Historical Society archives are a collection of articles and correspondence preserving the achievements of Bay Area–based activist, support worker, sex worker, and outreach advocate Tamara Ching (see fig. 2.4.). The archives documenting Ching's caregiving attest not merely to her individual achievements but to the collective impact of trans women's labor over time in demanding access to care. The now-historical local and national publications in this archive document the work of confronting multiple barriers that prevent trans women from accessing services. This archive calls into question why despite decades of labor by activists including Ching, many of these barriers remain in place today. Among these documents remains a single 8 × 11 sheet of white paper filled with large-font, Times New Roman type justified to fit the page. The note reads:

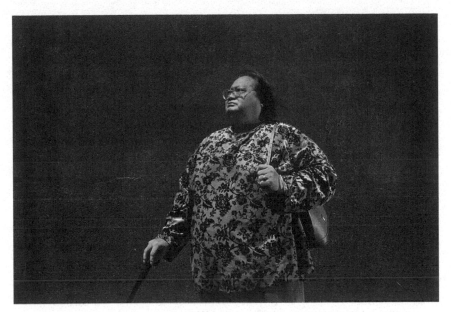

Figure 2.4. Portrait of trans HIV activist Tamara Ching. Printed with permission from Tamara Ching. Photo credit: Leah Millis/San Francisco Chronicle/Polaris.

please do not touch me
- i am being used by a
fat mean lady to try to
get hiv / aids services
for people being ig-
nored by the system.
she will be back in a
few minutes, **so don't
touch this.**
      signed,
      Miss U. No Huu

Included alongside this note are a series of articles, research studies, conference papers, and other print histories documenting Ching's legacy in advocating for the needs of trans women of color. Ching's archive addresses the struggles of trans women and their experiences of navigating housing and job discrimination, violence, economic barriers, sex work criminalization, and HIV, as those experiences intersect with one another and with racial and class-based oppression. Working with organizations including the Asian AIDS Project, the Gay Asian Pacific Alliance Community HIV Project (GCHP), the Transgender Services Coalition, and the San Francisco Human Rights Commission, Ching builds coalitions informed by her own experiences of facing employment barriers and of witnessing violence and death. She recalls her own experiences of surviving police harassment over decades as a sex worker in San Francisco's Tenderloin district. Ching traces her narratives back to the 1960s, when the neighborhood was the only space where trans women could congregate prior to the Compton Cafeteria Riots, which began a resistance movement in a claim to public space (Stryker, *Screaming Queens*). Ching also discusses the increasing challenges, since the 1960s, of surviving within a sex work economy wherein wages and working conditions continue to get worse for migrant women of color ("Stranger" 86). In mixing political mandate with humor, organizational research, and auto-biography, Ching's writing relates her own caregiving labor within trans self-determination movements to those directly addressing HIV.

Ching's autobiographical writing and activist work also narrates care as a collective endeavor. This collaborative work occurs at a community level to address individual access needs as connected to broader systems of gender-based violence. Rather than merely advocating for legal rights and inclusion, this work instead imagines transforming everyday acts of care that challenge rather than beg inclusion into state systems. The early HIV archive can therefore inspire present queer and trans movements to remove access barriers that affect all non-conforming bodies, rather than to focus politically on moving toward cultural assimilation and normativity. Returning now to Ching's archives offers a collective, community-centered model of caregiving activism that inspires antiassimilationist trans organizing today.

Gender Trash from Hell

This chapter's final section again revisits trans archives from the 1990s to connect the kinships formed in early responses to HIV to ongoing disability movements. The HIV kinships of the past offer narratives that resist state inclusion; instead, they demonstrate how trans caregiving can confront state systems that create medical inequalities, racism, and colonial violence. As Gill-Peterson reminds us, "*all* Western biomedicine continues to be eugenicist in practice, hoarding resources, stratifying quality of care, and normalizing the individual and population through high granular, racialized concepts of health that actively rely on a differential calculus of exhaustion, illness, and death for entire groups of people deemed undeserving" (*Histories* 199). In advocating for ongoing trans body self-determination through the archive, Gill-Peterson argues, a turn back to early trans medical narratives motivates an ongoing challenge to these systemic inequalities themselves. Trans HIV archives supporting such narratives include the Toronto-based do-it-yourself (DIY) zine *Gender Trash from Hell*. A DIY publication that "gives a voice to gender queers, who've been discouraged from speaking out & communicating with each other" (2), this zine again uses narrative production and distribution to reframe sites of body shame as creating collectivity. As Eichhorn argues, self-published zines and their preservation become a continuing intervention into the neoliberal destruction of small feminist presses (14–15). Extending on Eichhorn's work via *Gender Trash*, a return to the DIY, punk aesthetics of 1990s zine culture imagines a future that defies capitalist narratives enforcing cisgender body norms. The punk aesthetic of this publication is antiassimilationist in both its formal properties and its symbolic refusal to champion conformity to gender norms as a tactic for decreasing violence. Published from 1993 to 1995, *Gender Trash* is edited by Xanthra Mackay (under the name Xanthra Phillippa) with Mirha-Soleil Ross (under the pseudonym of Jeanne B.) acting as "Sexual & Political Advisor." *Gender Trash from Hell* introduces readers to the first issue with this poetic welcome:

> welcome gender queers
>> to the world of gender trash
>> our gender world
> where we can give voice
>> to our concerns in/around/about gender
>>> issues
>>> metamorphoses
>>> transformations
>>> changes
>>> loves
>>> lusts
>>> intensities
>>> hungers
>>> nightmares
>>> feelings about ourselves
>>> need to be valid on our own terms
>>>> to express ourselves in our own languages
>>>>> phrases
>>>>> words
>>>>> ways

This welcome continues for two more pages of the zine, outlining that the reader is being welcomed not just to a text but to a place wherein readers can come together to "move / glide freely / swarm / flock / herd / scream / shout / yell / fall / roll / crawl / ooze / slip / slide / play" (5). Mackay's welcome sets up trans writing (and self-publishing) as a forum through which to reimagine a future

> where we are not victims or victimized any longer
> a brand new world untouched by the Patriarchy & its horrors

a whole new beautiful world for us to explore

roam through
make love to

a world that is not owned by one

a few

a world that is shared by all of us
a world of our own
gender queers
please feel welcomed. (5)

Setting a poetic tone and space for trans expression as outside of capitalist patri-archy, the punk layout of the zine generates conversation with other 1990s movements and aesthetics. Returning to this zine's disability narratives offers ongoing anticapitalist models of queer and trans organizing that resist assimi-lation into gender and sexual norms.

The *Gender Trash* archive thus connects early HIV caregiving to the present by inspiring an ongoing resistance to medical narratives that pathologize bod-ies that do not conform. Like the trans women's archival newsletters and the writing of Ching, this first issue of *Gender Trash* positions disability access as a potential site of coalition building between trans and gay communities. This first issue showcases poetry, photography, art, and essays that address everything from terms and definitions to critiques of mainstream media, from safer elec-trolysis to "HERSTORY," from local resources to safer-sex information. These interconnected acts of care are all linked together and to issues of HIV and med-ical access (see fig. 2.5.). In a piece by Mackay, a full page of type set in individ-ual letter blocks reads, "TRANSSEXUALS / GET / AIDS / TOO / WHEN DO WE / GET NOTICED / THEIR LAUGHTER / IS KILLING US" (23). On the adjacent page, the reader is faced with a comparative chart. The left column reads, "This is what we have: ridicule / isolation / ignorance / hatred / no studies of our / own / no programs of our / own / no hospices of our / own / no support groups of our own" (24). In contrast, the right column presents a call to action: "This is what we need: no more ridicule / no more isolation / no more ignorance / no more hatred / studies of our own / programs of our own / hospices of our own / support groups of our own" (24). Responses to HIV reflect preexisting tensions between these two groups and position HIV caregiving as impetus to address existing structural inequalities. This piece again positions caregiving as that which can bring gay and trans organizers together by re-centering the access needs of those excluded by HIV movements.

Ross and Mackay also address these community rifts in their collaborative 1993 film *Gender Troublemakers*. The film presents an intimate portrait of Ross and Mackay's domestic relationship that cuts from shots of the lovers in bed to a series of documentary-style portraits wherein they take turns interviewing one

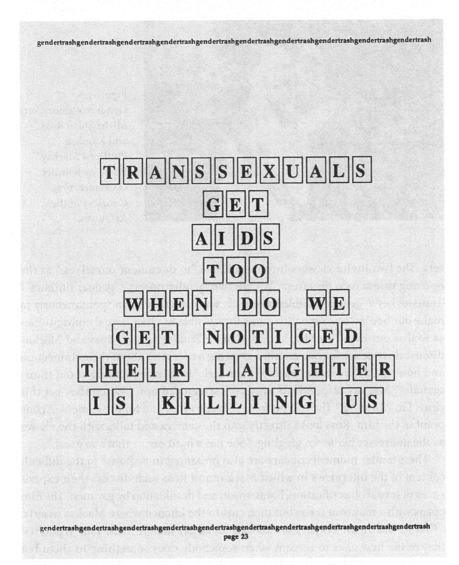

gendertrashgendertrashgendertrashgendertrashgendertrashgendertrashgendertrashgendertrashgendertrashgendertrash

TRANSSEXUALS
GET
AIDS
TOO
WHEN DO WE
GET NOTICED
THEIR LAUGHTER
IS KILLING US

gendertrashgendertrashgendertrashgendertrashgendertrashgendertrashgendertrashgendertrashgendertrashgendertrash
page 23

Figure 2.5. Art by Xanthra Phillippa Mackay from the debut issue of *Gender Trash from Hell* (1993). Courtesy of the ArQuives.

another in various locations in their home: in front of the kitchen counter, in front of a window, seated with a cat on a lap. The monochromatic pale yellows of the floral wallpaper and kitchen cabinets are offset by the vibrant 1990s fashion of the subjects. The film captures Ross in a black sports bra and Kelly-green overalls with thick vertical black stripes running down them, or in another bedroom scene Ross is completely naked and intertwined with Mackay, who remains (in some shots) fully clothed in layers of stern grey and black linen skirt

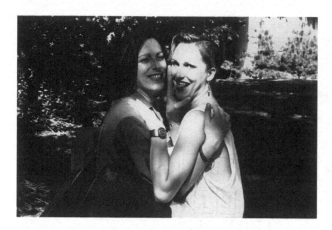

Figure 2.6.
Gendertroublemakers
Mirha Soleil Ross
and Xanthra
Phillippa Mackay.
Photo by Jennifer
O'Conner, 1993.
Courtesy of the
ArQuives.

sets. The two invite viewers into their home "to document ourselves," as the opening title screen declares, "We are two 'gender queers'/ 'gender outlaws' / 'trans-dykes' / 'gender troublemakers' . . . we made this video spontaneously to make our bodies, our sexualities, our lives visible to other sexual communities as well as our own." (see fig. 2.6.) In *Gender Troublemakers*, Ross and Mackay discuss their desire for one another, creating a narrative about their connection and how that desire makes each of them feel: "Is there something about transsexuals?" Mackay responds to Ross's off-screen prompt, "When they get this close, I'm vibrating." The two perform for each other and for the camera. At one point in the film, Ross looks directly into the camera and talks with the viewer as she undresses her lover, giggling: "She has a hard on . . . that's so great."

These tender moments of care are also presented in response to the difficult content of the interviews in which Mackay and Ross each discuss their experiences of sexual objectification, harassment, and devaluation by gay men. The film opens with a makeout scene but then cuts to the kitchen where Mackay asserts, "This is what really bothers me about a lot of gay men, is their real hypocrisy, they're the first ones to scream when somebody does something to them but they have no problems about being very discriminating and being very prejudiced and very creepy to other groups, other disadvantaged, groups such as us." Mackay testifies to how gay male community has been "anything but supportive. I feel like I am on display, I've always felt that. As a freakshow." Mackay recounts,

> As soon as I started wearing skirts and dresses, my sex life dropped to as near as zero. . . . And I was really pissed off at that because people would say, well, I guess you're going to have to make a decision between wearing skirts and getting sex. And I was really upset because it wasn't a decision I could make: I was expressing myself at something I had to do. And the idea that I was going

to lose out . . . it just really upset me. At the same time, I just said, well, this is more important than getting laid all the time. . . . [The men] were not worth it anyways. . . . They weren't worth rearranging my life to fit them. So I just said fine, forget it, they weren't all that hot in bed anyways.

The film then presents a sex scene between the pair, offsetting the rejection of gay community with the connection of trans women loving each other. This film's discussion in 1993 of violence against trans women within gay spaces within HIV organizing remains salient into the present. Returning to these critiques today offers a narrative of the past that is neither heroic nor complete, opening space to continue this labor of increasing trans resources, improving coalitions, and breaking isolation. Alexandra Juhasz and Ted Kerr's work looks backward to HIV archives not to narrate a static history but to understand how such narratives of the past inform experiences of HIV as ongoing. Juhasz and Kerr critique the 2013 Hollywood film *Dallas Buyers Club* in order to show how current representations of HIV create false stories about the "pastness of HIV" by inaccurately portraying HIV narratives as already resolved. Connecting early HIV archives with younger generations continuing to fight for queer and trans access resists creating a linear progression from past to present. Instead, revisiting these works inspires a temporally queer narrative model that cuts across time and space to continue to form caregiving kinships in response to disability.

These archives are thus helpful not merely as records of a past moment but as inspiring ongoing kinships for resisting body norms. Like *Gender Troublemakers*, *Gender Trash* imagines its readership as a queer and trans community that can coalesce in response to the personal narratives the zine presents. The authors address gaps in medical access by identifying areas where coalition building fails. This archive, accordingly, demonstrates the impact of caregiving in addressing the isolation and stigma caused at the intersections of gender-based and medical violence. For instance, in the third issue of *Gender Trash* in 1995, Mackay includes the poem "Don't Touch Me—I'm Electric TS Epileptic," which shares her experience of seeking support for epilepsy within both trans and medical communities. Her piece discusses doctors' reductive treatment of Mackay's trans identity as well as the medical industry's broader marginalization of trans-ness by labeling trans identity as a medical side effect of epilepsy treatment. She critiques the "Pure Ableist Middle Class TS Fantasy Land," wherein doctors reduce trans identity to the result of seizure medication, and where trans communities present access barriers for disabled people. Because her critique takes the form of poetry, it engages readers in her experience both on a practical and on an emotional level, sharing how isolation is felt in the absence of care. Poetry operates differently than other types of community-centered writing in that it performs the speaker's experience for the readers to take up collectively:

So I guess I don't belong to the True Transsexual Community
        because the community for which I have been searching for
                is one that would welcome me
                        & others like me
                            as we are
                                without hesitation

While Mackay's earlier entries on HIV begin to demonstrate rifts between trans and gay communities, this piece expands the narrative process of addressing community fractures in order to improve chosen family models of care. The poem's opening line, "I found out I'm not a real transsexual anymore," is both reactive and direct, outlining the difficulty of holding one's self-determined embodiments against the authority of clinical narratives. Although the statement implies dismissive critique through its sarcasm, it also candidly confronts the feelings of defeat and of urgency surrounding the medical system's diagnostic power, as well as corresponding community barriers to valuing disability. In conversation with this chapter's range of HIV archives, this trans disability narrative offers ongoing strategies for processing medical trauma by continuing to create welcoming spaces where trans bodies need not align with able-bodied norms.

This chapter revisits early HIV archives to re-center narratives of the often-invisible gendered labor that brings communities together in response to disability. While these archives from the 1980s and 1990s hold the potential to imagine more-caring futures, the HIV archiving process itself reinforces original CDC definitions of AIDS that exclude trans women and erase gendered experiences of HIV. However, in preserving trans women's caregiving legacies through collections of gender troublemakers and safer-sex workshops, community newsletters, and memorial interviews, these archives attest to strategies for increasing disability access through the formation of anticapitalist, antiassimilationist HIV kinships. These narratives of assembling chosen families inspire an analysis of fictional and autobiographical writing in chapter 3, which places the early HIV family narratives of Sarah Schulman and Iris De La Cruz in conversation with the contemporary trans writing of Bryn Kelly and Casey Plett. Chapter 3 takes up a further investigation of how the failures of biological family inspire queer and trans chosen families in order to meet caregiving needs. In creating disability kinships while also documenting failures in receiving adequate support, trans women's archives offset medical narratives to better care for bodies that do not conform.

Chosen Families

REJECTION, DESIRE, AND ARCHIVES OF CARE

Upon entering the hospital as a sex worker with AIDS symptoms in the 1980s, Iris De La Cruz was denied access to care. The solution to this medical mistreatment, De La Cruz recalls, was found in her mother: "I have seen my mother physically drag a nurse into my room to take care of me. Residents used to hide out in the medication room when they heard my mother was on the floor." De La Cruz's HIV narratives provide a range of possibilities for reimagining disability via the family. De La Cruz's writing offers caregiving models that blend biological and chosen family, a narrative strategy central to the contemporary trans fiction of Casey Plett. Extending from my analysis of trans archives in chapter 2, I revisit De La Cruz's archives to observe how early HIV family formations continue to influence queer and trans caregiving kinships. While chapter 1 imagines interdependence through vampire fiction and safer-sex archives, and chapter 2 uncovers the administrative and caregiving labor of building coalitions, this chapter draws on fiction and autobiography to narrate HIV through chosen family formations.

In revisiting this same historical moment in New York City as De La Cruz's work, I begin this chapter by looking back to Sarah Schulman's 1995 novel *Rat Bohemia*, which represents HIV as the result of not viral pathology but parental cruelty. Schulman's queer characters exhibit a variety of emotional and physical symptoms in response to homophobia and gender correction from their parents. I move from this investigation of Schulman's HIV fiction to an analysis of Sur Rodney (Sur)'s oral history of creating Visual AIDS in response to familial neglect. Jumping from this past back into the present, I consider this formation of queer and trans chosen family within Bryn Kelly's HIV *Partybottom* Tumblrs and fiction and Plett's contemporary short fiction to connect current disability communities to these earlier narratives of HIV kinship. This chapter then returns again to early HIV narratives to revisit the caregiving archives of De La Cruz. I read these texts all together across genres, media, and time to consider how early HIV narratives continue to inspire queer and trans family formations for gender self-determination. Through these HIV narratives, disability is reframed not as an individual or pathological problem but as powerful in generating chosen family when biological kin fail to care.

FAMILY TROUBLE

This section returns to literary and archival HIV narratives to offer models of chosen family that continue to inspire disability kinships into the present. Schulman's HIV fiction narrates physical suffering not merely as an outcome of illness but as a breakdown in the biological family's capacities for support. Responding to these gaps in care, Schulman's work also represents the chosen families that emerge in response to family harm. As an activist, writer, and member of ACT UP/New York, Schulman was one of the first novelists to publish fiction representing lesbians and HIV. In Schulman's *Rat Bohemia*, the lesbian heroine, Rita, and her gay co-narrator, David, trace the associations between familial abandonment and the progression of illness. The two concur, "There is nothing on earth that could kill us more efficiently than parental indifference" (63). David connects the emergence of his own AIDS symptoms to his family's refusal to accept "little courageous sissy-wissy me" with "limp wrists and a will of steel" (64). His feelings of rejection mirror Rita's frustration that in trying to elicit love from her father, "[she] always get[s] destroyed" (189). She lists the tangible symptoms of abandonment by her biological family: "feeling sick to my stomach, ugly, hateful, repulsive, disgusting . . . knowing that I am bad" (188). Schulman's fiction responds to historically entrenched medical narratives that position homosexuality as an inevitable cause of physical decline (Long 30; Román, *Acts of Intervention* xxi; Edelman 81; Denneny 42; Nunokawa 311; Bordowitz, *AIDS Crisis* 66; "Surviving the AIDS Genocide"; McGrath and Sutcliffe 9; Love 6; Hoppe 2). In the 2003 foreword to the debut issue of the now-archival HIV publication *Corpus*, George Ayala reflects, "One of the great ironies of the AIDS era (or perhaps logical outcome) is the inordinate attention given to understanding the biology of HIV in the body without regard to the bodies hosting the virus" (vii). *Corpus* uncovers how cultural narratives of HIV are informed by epidemiologists, doctors, and scientists. Outlining the capacities for cultural production to intervene in pathologizing, anti-queer medical narratives (Hebert x), *Corpus* editor Jamie Cortez declares, "I like this part of the HIV response spectrum. I like it because I want to learn of new strains of faggotry. I like it because I want to see queer male life strategies transmitted and reproduced with virulence. I want pathology reports, Miss Thing. I want to know we're present even when undetectable. I want us to survive in the millions" (xi). Cultural production, Schulman's fiction also demonstrates, counters such narratives that justify parental cruelty toward queer and trans children under the auspice of protecting them from harm (*Ties* 2009; Spurlin 92). This narrative process can also be found in family storytelling practices that render disabled children as unlovable because of their disabilities (Erickson, "Revealing" 42–43). In contesting these medical narratives through HIV fiction, these archives reposition family trouble as caused by homophobia and cissexism (and not homosexuality and trans-ness). HIV archives likewise identify how ableism (and not disability) is the problem in need of a cure.

Early HIV narratives, accordingly, offer an ongoing model for narrating disability differently through representations of HIV kinships. *Rat Bohemia* demonstrates how barriers to receiving support from biological family motivate queer caregiving networks in response to HIV. Schulman uses fiction to position the cause of David's suffering from AIDS not with symptoms of his illness but with his family. Schulman's novels frame the family (support systems) and not the sick body (disabled individuals) as requiring intervention. Derailing the narrative that locates the disabled body as the source of trauma, David tells the reader about the cause of his terminal condition: "I realized that my parents were trying to kill me. In fact, my entire family is in on it. . . . My father's favorite tactic for killing me is to never call. . . . Occasionally my parents go on vacation and I'll get a postcard signed MOM. Or a birthday card signed MOM. He's killing me, my dad. He obviously wants me to die" (63). While the chapter's introduction to this phenomenon of parents killing their children through a lack of kindness initially seems perhaps melodramatic, as the chapter progresses, it switches from sarcasm to realism to revisit flashbacks of parental cruelty from David's childhood. David recounts, "As a child I was always being gender-corrected. I was one of those little boys with a high squeaky voice who waved his hands in the air and got too excited. It made my parents deeply uncomfortable. . . . There was always an invisible Dave, one that had never existed and could never exist, that they expected to find miraculously each morning at the breakfast table. And when, instead, all they got was little silly-willy me . . . they were deeply angry" (64). In fictionalizing this parental anger in response to gender self-determination, Schulman's literary reimagining of disability shifts the onus away from the sick body and onto the family as the object of scrutiny in need of correction.

David's narrative therefore transfers the origin story of his illness away from his individual body and onto his family. This narrative shift is significant in representing disability as connected to caregiving breakdowns in institutions like the family rather than as merely a product of individual pathology. In a childhood flashback to a "cold winter's Sunday back in 1968" (63), David recounts an incident through which his brother and sister "were recruited" (65) by his parents to "learn how to kill" (65). David recalls driving through "the winter stillness" (64) along "incomprehensible country byways" (64) with his family. This pastoral setting becomes the backdrop to this now frozen-in-time moment of David's being commanded out of the car and "out into the snow" (64) for disagreeing with his father about "the fun of getting lost" (64). David recounts being "just a little boy" (64) and standing on the asphalt alone, watching his family's car drive away without him. Though expected to run after the car as it idles just ahead up the one-way road, returning to his family "humiliated . . . and most importantly, quiet" (64), David instead continues to walk away from the car in the opposite direction, "soberly, with determination" (65). David thus forces his family to retrace their path "back along the same route from the beginning" (65) in order to pick him back up again.

David's determined rerouting of the cis het family trajectory also offers the potential to expand the family's norms toward reincorporating their queer child. David imagines this process as one of collaboration in which his departure could bring greater cohesion to the family by inspiring the combined effort of all remaining members. He recounts, "I . . . pictured the four of them rationally dissecting the map, trying to efficiently reach their goal, which was me" (65). However, rather than actualizing this fantasy, David "plopped" (65) himself back into the car only to be "greeted" (65) by the "sheer terror" (65) on his siblings' faces: "their fear of my experience was to have a much more profound effect on their lives than the experience they dreaded had actually had on mine" (65). Drawing from this childhood flashback, David presents his experience of HIV stigma as directly connected to his family's early and continued rendering of his differences as grounds for exclusion. David's HIV narrative can be connected to broader cultural narratives that render disabled bodies as inassimilable and feared for their inability to conform to definitions of "normal" (Garland-Thomson 45). The fears underlying HIV stigma, this flashback suggests, indicate a problem inherent not to disability or to bodies living with HIV but to institutions like David's family that fail to map out routes that value difference.

Rat Bohemia thus offers a narrative model for using storytelling to reverse medical narratives that blame individuals for social problems. Such strategies toward destigmatizing HIV in particular and disability more broadly can begin with the family. David exposes this tendency to regard disability as a medical rather than social problem. He ponders this phenomenon by challenging media narratives of cures for HIV: "Why didn't the newspapers announce . . . that parental kindness helps people with AIDS live longer? Because that's asking for more than people can do. Love our gay children? Impossible! We just want a pill, it's easier" (53). This narrative shift from individual biomedical narratives onto social family narratives occurs in other queer HIV fiction from this period, including lesbian writer Patricia Powell's 1994 HIV novel, *A Small Gathering of Bones*. In Powell's narrative, which follows the relationships of queer men in Jamaica responding to HIV in the early years of the pandemic, the hero Dale's best friend Ian's experience of disability is connected to his devastating rejection by his own mother for being gay. When Dale puts his faith in medical doctors to save his dying friend, Ian's sister exclaims, "But Dale, she push him" (134), recounting the culpability of their mother's violent expulsion of her son as the equally probable cause of his suffering. Such narrative strategies reframe disability as motivating critiques of larger systems for causing individual body harm; narrative becomes a tool for connecting suffering to limits in caregiving from family but also in connecting larger systemic factors including racism and colonialism that prevent families from being able to care for queer and trans kin. As trans advocate Janet Mock identifies in her autobiography *Redefining Realness*, even when parents are unconditionally loving toward their children, multiple barriers might still prevent caregivers from effectively providing support: "Not all trans people come of age in supportive middle- and upper-middle-class homes where parents have resources and access to knowledgeable and affordable health care" (119). Mock further discusses how the media's representation of high-income white families accessing trans-affirming health care for their children erases the existence of trans communities of color and issues they face, including barriers to health-care access (119). By shifting the story away from individuals' bodies and toward interventions in institutions, HIV fiction offers a caregiving critique of the family toward increasing accessibility and destigmatizing difference. Early HIV narratives document this process of creating disability kinships that continue to address structural barriers to accessing family care.

SUCH TIGHT, CLOSE FRIENDS

This next section shifts from an analysis of fiction to revisit oral histories documenting early HIV caregiving in response to the failures of biological families. Narratives of HIV-chosen family respond to gaps in care and can continue to inspire disability kinships. These early HIV kinships are preserved within archives commemorating the organizational history of the New York City–based organization Visual AIDS. In a blog post, Visual AIDS recalls its own history of forming in response to family failures: "Many artists were spending thirty or forty percent of their time dealing with HIV/AIDS related concerns. . . . Many stopped creating new works, and, as they were dying and after their deaths the work they had accomplished was lost, thrown out, or forgotten." This blog attests to the historical prevalence of this problem of preservation: "People's families would come and just throw things out. . . . It was real. It was terrifying. . . . It just broke my heart." The authors recirculate a "darkly funny" zine that "features a trashcan complete with an accompanying sewer rat. The text across the can spells out 'life's work.' It is captioned, 'His name was Robert, cutest boy in the East Village—someone said. Molto Talento (Great Animal Sculpture) Now Landfill.'" The blog traces this experience of loss in which people who were sick would also have to worry about what would happen to their art when they died. The work of Visual AIDS demonstrates how archiving as a process creates chosen family by bringing people together through this act of artistic preservation.

Early HIV histories also leverage the archive itself to preserve these legacies and transmit these material histories across generations. In an oral history interview for the Smithsonian's *Archives of American Art*, Ted Kerr interviews Sur, a prominent black gay gallery owner who ran Gracie Mansion Gallery (with collaborator Gracie Mansion) in the East Village in the 1980s. Sur recounts leaving the gallery to provide full-time care to people living with HIV in his neighborhood who were abandoned by their biological families. Using his skills in curation and art dealership, Sur discusses how he begins archiving the art of the community members with whom he exchanges care. Sur's narrative demonstrates the impact of his caregiving labor in forming HIV kinships. He characterizes his caregiving role as one of confronting disability stigma. Sur recounts spending increasing amounts of time with people who needed care, including his neighbors, friends, lovers, and even strangers in the hospital who were often there alone. He remembers a critical moment while visiting Keith Davis, an artist "critically important in the whole East Village thing," during a period while Davis was feeling isolated:

> He had a really difficult time, and I kind of felt that he needed support. Not so much in terms of helping to do things, because he wasn't that ill yet, and he had a good support system, but he really needed like more of the emotional support. So I would do things. And I remember inviting him here over to dinner one day, and he came over, and I cooked this meal, and he ate some of it and left it on his plate, and then I started like finishing the food that was on his plate. And he just froze, because he thought of himself as such a pariah that the idea that I had no problem with eating the food off of his plate, thinking to himself, "nothing like that has ever happened to me before." It was really kind of like this amazing thing that happened to him. It was like for a moment in his life, in all these weeks that he'd been going through this, for the first time he didn't feel like his infection really mattered, and that's when I—just from that interchange—from that moment on, I'd realized a lot of what these people are going through not only . . . [means they] have to negotiate through their day to day but [also negotiate] just their feeling about themselves.

This "interchange" acknowledges the notion that caregiving includes not merely help "to do things" but also "emotional support," and as Sur recounts, sex: "We were lovers for a while. And I was lovers with him, I think, either right before he'd had his diagnosis, or he'd already been diagnosed, and to me, it didn't matter." Sur also depicts joining caregiver support groups and attending memorials of friends, which brought him closer to other caregivers to become "such tight, close friends." He relays how at the support groups "most of the caregivers that came through are mostly white and mostly men. Most—pretty much gay. And a lot of them were trying to have sex with me. [Laughs.] I mean, the whole thing was going on with the sex thing in hospitals with doctors and caregivers was really—that a whole other sort of sordid story." Sur's narrative frames caregiving as holding the potential, even in medical spaces, to create lasting kinships through friendship, care, and sex. These narratives of caregiving-as-intimacy are also evidenced by archival testimonies from a variety of HIV caregivers including Debbie Warren, a lesbian minister who founded the Regional AIDS Interfaith Network (RAIN) in South Carolina to organize faith-based HIV caregiving teams within religious communities. In a 2014 audio installation by Jessica Whitbread, Warren records the history of forming RAIN, describing how the type of care RAIN provides is "not nursing care, but friendship, companionship." Warren recalls how "lots of people who were very sick with AIDS lived much longer than they were predicted to live because they had these loving people around them." While the inclusion of sex into spaces of care is often narrated as potentially creating harm, the sex cultures in Sur's narrative counter the isolation attached to disability by instead centering the potential of forming caregiving connections toward countering sexual stigma (Erickson, "Revealing" 42). Sites of care are rendered through the early HIV archives as a locus of HIV community formation. Bringing this disability archive into the present continues to model caregiving as facilitating queer and trans kinships, emotional connections, and sex.

Sur's narrative also frames these acts of care as transformative in creating chosen families in response to disability. For Sur, such kinships included preserving the art of people living with HIV. Sur recounts how he used to say, "Whenever I meet an artist that is really energetic and really prolific and really determined to grind out a lot of work, they're probably living with AIDS." Sur traces the progression through which his day-to-day caregiving practice also became one of archiving and collection: "I ended up acquiring a lot of material from a lot of these artists because they were afraid that it wouldn't be protected, and they knew that I would protect it. So that went on for a number of years and became exhausted. . . . I was becoming like, really like, what do I do with all the stuff." Sur's work brought him into contact with other caregivers in his community including Frank Moore who were doing the same type of curatorial care, and together they began building the archive that is now Visual AIDS. For Sur, curating became a form of community formation and of activism that was more accessible for him than street protests with ACT UP. As a black man from Montreal who was living in the United States without status, Sur found himself avoiding getting arrested but instead undertaking caregiving activism in ways he found particularly impactful. Revisiting his work reveals how much his "single body" was able to do in exchanging care with friends, lovers, neighbors, and strangers, assembling an archive of HIV-chosen family creation. Kerr's interview with Sur brings these early HIV activisms into contemporary representation to inspire ongoing queer and trans models of care. Like Schulman's fictional account of addressing biological family failures, Sur's narratives continue to inspire ongoing disability kinships into the present, including the archiving and remembering of these histories themselves.

You Have Become a Cyborg God/dess

This section moves from this print archive into the present to consider how digital HIV narratives continue to create chosen family through their online readership and distribution. While Schulman's fiction identifies the impact of bio-logical family failures, and Sur's archives attest to the formation of chosen family in preserving the art of people living with HIV, contemporary disability narra-tives continue to inspire caregiving in response to HIV. Schulman and Sur's archives can be read as connected to an ongoing legacy of queer and trans HIV narratives like those found online in *Partybottom: The *Sexy* HIV+ Transgen-der Blog* (partybottom.tumblr.com), which Kelly updated from 2013 to 2015. Kelly, a trans New York City–based artist, writer, and activist living with HIV, died at age thirty-five in 2016 (see fig. 3.1.). Kelly's legacy is memorialized in her online writing which addresses a wide range of practical issues for navigating health-care access and social service systems. Her *Partybottom* blog creates a family of readers who write to her for advice. Kelly's Tumblr guides her readers through the harsh daily realities of navigating "the HIV Welfare Merry-Go Round," an endless turnover of case workers, queer and trans collective housing, and other "institutional problems that lead to trans women getting bad care." In a post from August 18, 2014, Kelly discusses how in queer HIV service organizations, "trans women are systematically shut out of the process of decision-making around HIV prevention and education." Kelly identifies how such organizations lump together their clients living with HIV "including 'trans women and men who have sex with men,' in one breath, populations that have historically been blurred together, often to the detriment of trans women's ability to access services." Kelly also discusses the hiring practices in these institutions as erroneously favoring education over life experience. In a post dated December 13, 2013, she writes, "If you prioritize education and being able to speak a certain kind of social-work-y, tenderqueer vernacular, you will get providers who can provide services for white, FAAB [female assigned at birth], transmasculine people. If you prioritize hiring people from the communities you hope to serve—people who have *lived the life*—you will serve those communities, and, hopefully, serve them well." Relatedly, in her post from August 18, 2014, Kelly discusses the tendency of queer community organizations to prioritize the hiring of social workers who iden-tify as queer and/or as transmasculine over social workers (queer and straight) who have dedicated their lives to understanding how to navigate the systems their trans women clients must access. Kelly recalls one particularly transfor-mative experience with such a social worker, reflecting, "When I am her age, she is who I want to be. God bless her." The support Kelly provides for other trans

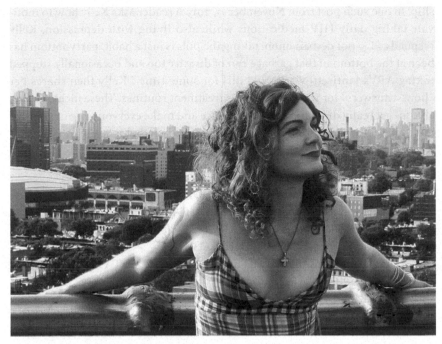

Figure 3.1. Photograph of Bryn Kelly by Julian Talamantez Brolaski, 2013. Photo credit: Julian Talamantez Brolaski.

women navigating these services is framed through narrative accounts of her own vulnerable feelings. Kelly presents painful content in tandem with camp cheer and fun, always ending her posts with "something magical." For instance, at the end of her entry from August 1, 2014 about having to pointlessly spend full days in welfare offices applying for disability programs she knows she will repeatedly be rejected from,[1] Kelly observes the "solidarity" formed between herself and others forced through the system: "We make small talk. We encourage each other. We share advice about what we have learned about the system. We make sure that we are taken care of. In small, understated, undramatic ways, we show each other tiny acts of love. And there is beauty in that" (2014).

The countless "tiny acts of love" with which Kelly provides care are commemorated throughout her writing. Many of Kelly's Tumblr posts contain autobiographical narratives, memes, reblogs from other trans women living with HIV, and photos of her daily medicine regimes as color-coordinated with her nail polish or as accompanied by enticing imagery of her home-cooked omelets. Kelly also answers "asks," responding to the comments and questions of her reader-

---

1. Kelly hashtags this experience: "#kafka-esque bureaucracy." This hashtag is not very functional but remains helpful nevertheless.

ship. In one such post from November 17, 2015, a reader asks Kelly how to motivate taking daily HIV medications while also living with depression. Kelly responds, "Do not despair anon! taking the pills is just a habit. partybottom has been at the bottom of that garbage can of disaster too and occasionally stopped taking ARVs [antiretroviral cocktails] for some time." Kelly then shares her "honest answers" for why she practices treatment routines. These include being able to "get really dramatic about adherence and make everyone else in your life miserable complaining about it which sucks for them but is really fun for you." Kelly also encloses an all-caps list of her "final" and "most important" advice:

—YOU HAVE TIGER BLOOD AND ADONIS DNA—
—YOU HAVE BECOME A CYBORG GOD/DESS—
—YOU ARE EVOLVED BEYOND THE GRASP OF A MERE VIRUS
    THAT HAS CLAIMED THE LIVES OF 39 MILLION PEOPLE—
—YOU ARE THE GHOST IN THE MACHINE—
—YOU ARE THE BASTARD STEP DAUGHTER OF STATE SOCIALISM
    AND GLOBAL CAPITALISM—
—YOU ARE NEW PHARMACOPORNOGRAPHIC REGIME—
—YOU—
—HAVE—
—T I G E R—
—B L O O D—

The post is accompanied by a photo of a red blood droplet with tiger stripes on it, and the words "Tiger Blood" flanking it (a pop culture reference to Charlie Sheen's self-reported resilience to recreational drug use). This post presents a paradigm shift based on hybridity and animacy that reframes reliance on medication as transformative (and playful) rather than merely as pathological. In linking the individual body living with HIV to larger systems of god/desses, cyborgs, pharmaceuticals, and global capitalism, Kelly both brings levity to difficult problems and validates the weight of daily responsibility for dealing with the embodied consequences of larger social systems. Kelly's Tumblr further discusses her own experience with biomedical judgment and surveillance, which she works through with her readers, in her writing. In a post dated May 30, 2014, she reflects on being mistrusted about her medical adherence by her doctors, and about being "undetectable" which she reflects "is cool and all, but 'undetectable' is imho kind of bullshit, if for no other reason than they keep moving the target." In a post on her personal blog (brynkelly.tumblr.com) from December 2, 2013, Kelly also debates her feelings about pre-exposure prophylaxis (PrEP) with other Tumblr writers including Morgan M. Page, arguing that she is happy that people have the choice whether or not to take it despite its connection to regimes of control and surveillance. As Simone Browne argues in her critical analysis of blackness and surveillance, "dark matter is that nonluminous component of the universe that is said to exist but cannot be observed, cannot be re-created in laboratory conditions. Its distribution cannot be measured; its properties cannot be determined; and so it remains undetectable" (9). Undetectability, identifies Browne, illuminates how antiblack racism and surveillance are "practiced, narrated, and enacted" (9). In tracing these concepts of undetectability through medical surveillance, Kelly also identifies the state mechanisms through which biomedical narratives further pathologize bodies living with HIV. Her writing thus builds a readership of chosen family by representing new approaches for narrating undetectability and disability kinships.

In addition to writing for people living with HIV, Kelly also addresses audiences of seronegative queer and trans readers to provide her communities with education on how to care for chosen family members who are living with HIV. As such, Kelly's blog intends to build family support systems between seronegative and seropositive members of queer and trans communities. Kelly's 2014 article "How to Be a Good Roommate to Someone Living with HIV/AIDS" was commissioned by the Trans Housing Network (a Tumblr network "intended to connect trans people in need with safe and supportive places to crash") and circulated across various social media platforms including Facebook. In her article, Kelly outlines the disjuncture between the antioppressive politics lip serviced within queer and trans rhetoric and the actual practices of discrimination faced by people living with HIV in queer and trans communities. She conjures a hypothetical "housing ad on Craigslist. $400 room available, must like cats, queer/trans friendly house!" She then details the selection process during which people living with HIV might make themselves vulnerable in a roommate interview by disclosing their HIV status and housing access needs, only to be rejected in favor of an applicant who is seronegative and not facing similar barriers. "Who would you choose?" poses Kelly: "This is where the social justice rubber hits the road." Kelly discusses these potential access needs in detail, familiarizing readers with both the institutional and personal challenges for which people living with HIV rely on their roommates' support rather than further housing discrimination.

Drawing on her personal experiences with queer and trans collective living, Kelly also instructs readers on how to provide better care to their chosen families. She emphasizes in all-caps, "IT IS NO ONE'S RIGHT TO DISCLOSE ANYONE'S HIV STATUS BUT THEIR OWN." Kelly appeals to readers' prior understanding of *outing* and discrimination, comparing HIV disclosure to safety issues of gender passing: "There is a real parallel here with being trans. Some trans people are OUT OUT OUT about being trans—and that's great!—and other people are super stealth and don't want anyone to know about it. It is sort of the same with HIV." Kelly draws on community language, referencing understood paradigms of what it means to be "OUT OUT OUT" or "super stealth" to reinforce how HIV disclosure is a matter of self-determination. Kelly draws on her own life narratives to provide examples of how well-intentioned housemates

have disclosed her HIV status simply by talking about how she relies on sources
of income from HIV social programs to pay her share of the rent:

> Say your roommate seems not to be doing much. Like, if they are caught up
> in the HIV/AIDS industrial complex, they are probably consigned to a life of
> subsistence poverty, so it is likely that they may have a little side hustle to afford
> things that most normal people have (like, say, a cell phone! or shoes that don't
> hurt your feet! or whatever!) Maybe they cut hair for cash. Maybe they deal a
> little weed. Maybe they work under the table at a food truck. Maybe they play
> music and busk on the train. Odds are, they may have a life that appears
> improbable to the outside world.

In counseling readers on strategies of how not to disclose a roommate's HIV status, Kelly also writes in support of lives that are "improbable" under able-
bodied, capitalist definitions of labor and worth. "There is dignity in just being,"
Kelly writes in a poetic Tumblr post dated May 29, 2014; "your life is worth living even if you're 'not doing anything.'" Kelly also addresses the right of people
living with HIV to self-determine if and when they choose to discuss their status to their sexual partners: "People living with HIV know better than anyone
else the right time and place and circumstance to disclose matters of their own
health. This is not your job." Kelly discusses the stigma faced by people living
with HIV who can be treated by their queer and trans family like "'AIDS monsters' who run around trying to infect people at every given opportunity." Kelly
reminds readers, "both my IRL [In Real Life] experience and all the public health
data do not bear this out. (Most new infections are between people who do not
know their status.)"

Kelly's writing ultimately identifies the critical role of roommates as caregivers for one another and the importance of being "a good friend." Extending caregiver possibilities beyond just parents and partners—types of nuclear family
support not available for all queer and trans people—Kelly's writing expands
models of family by detailing the impact of domestic and community support:
"Life with HIV can feel lonely and sad sometimes," Kelly shares. "Depression is
always kind of knocking on your door. Lots of people—HIV+ and HIV-—feel
this way, and everyone copes with this differently—and having nice friends
around to shoot the shit with over a cup of tea or a beer is a great coping mechanism." In giving the advice to "maybe be a buddy" and accompany a roommate
to an appointment or to pay more of the rent if one is financially able—a system
Kelly connects to Rivera and Johnson's 1970s trans housing projects like STAR—
Kelly frames caregiving as a domestic act that develops chosen family. She concludes: "The main take away is this: as queers, we need to take seriously our com-
mitments to caring for one another. It is not always easy. It *can* be fun. But it
is crucial. It is how we survive. It is how we have always survived" (Kelly).

This struggle with survival and with chosen family is also central to Kelly's fictional writing. In "Other Balms, Other Gileads," a short story published in *We Who Feel Differently* (2014), these daily acts of self-care and queer and trans domestic negotiations are represented through Kelly's haunting prose. We follow a day in the life of the story's trans narrator as she goes grocery shopping, worries about her new subletter, cooks dinner for her trans boyfriend, gives him a blow job, negotiates his expectations for constant sex from her (even while she is cooking), and supports him (again) in filling out his application for PrEP, a conversation that "reminds her of the toxicity flowing through her veins, filling her spine, and seeping from between her legs." The narrator's boyfriend (who spends the day watching porn in the narrator's bed and dabbling in some graduate school work) talks about how the drug will alleviate their fears of HIV transmission, even though, as the narrator identifies, "the way they have sex now, the risk of his being infected must be something like the odds of being hit by lightning. Or winning the lottery." The story thus cycles back to its own beginning where the opening lines place the narrator at the store while she waits to use her food stamps, watching the cashier sell lottery tickets and remembering things "her liberal friends say about gambling." These meditations on probability and risk emphasize the disjuncture between the care the narrator takes of her boyfriend and the ways he frames her body as being "wounded." She discloses her history of surviving sexual violence, musing: "A diagnosis of HIV comes with very few blessings, but in this instance it was, for her, a measure of safety. A sign that said, *Do not come near. Biohazardous.* Barbed wire and guard dogs." In working through the meanings of the pleasure she receives from this boyfriend, she interprets his insatiable desire for her body as a threat to the care she tries to provide: "She knows he is edging. She has food on the stove and it could burn and he is using her mouth like a toy, taking his sweet time. She has always had an affinity for pump-and-dump guys; she sees delayed orgasm as something for tweekers and other degenerates (she knows a lot about tweekers and degenerates.) She wants to be fucked like dogs fuck—a few thrusts, then cum, then a knot to tie the two animals together to give them time to imprint on each other, and then to be done with it." Because the food "could burn" without the pair leaving any "imprint on each other," the narrative consistently displays how there remains no correlation between the amount of care the narrator sinks into the connection and the strength of the connection itself. Instead, the boyfriend challenges the narrator's decisions regarding her own medication choices, undermining her self-knowledge and judging her drug use (the narrator discusses with us her addiction to a variety of mail order prescription pills to deal with her anxiety after receiving disrespectful care from her own clinicians). The narrator spends a great deal of the story attempting to understand the connections between her body's limits and pharmaceuticals' promise of salvation: "Did this disease shatter her somewhere along the way, and she didn't even notice it? Is she gulping down these chunky robin's-egg-colored compounds every morning because they promise to fill the chunk of her heart that's missing?" Extending on *Rat Bohemia*'s prescription for parental kindness and *Partybottom*'s vision of roommate support, our "cyber god/dess" narrator ponders the limits of biomedical technology and gendered domestic inequality as sources of care.

Kelly's work thus raises caregiving considerations that reanimate early HIV archives in the present. By reading Kelly's family trouble as forming a narrative lineage with Schulman and Sur, these early HIV narratives offer ongoing kinship models in support of sexual and gender self-determination. In "Sharps Container Ghosts," his 2014 review essay on "Other Balms, Other Gileads," Doug Keeler analyzes Kelly's short story alongside his examination of the "AIDS Crisis Revisitations," contemporary mainstream films that have been critiqued by scholars including Juhasz and Kerr for their historically inaccurate centering of the achievements of white men and for framing HIV as something that remains in the distant past ("Home Video"). Such retellings of HIV history, Keeler explains, employ a narrative tactic that "transparently taps into the universality of death and loss, but also the overwhelming sentimentality of homophobia." Keeler considers why a generation of people who were not present during this period in HIV history get "so worked up about" these films. Keeler elaborates: "The Revisitation invokes a more complex affective tension for the HAART [Highly Active Antiretroviral Therapy] generation (queers coming of age after the introduction of antiretroviral therapy around 1996): a sense of orphanage, of having our would-be genealogy severed. These films and performances are sad because they remind us that the people who could have taught us how to fuck and how to love are long dead. Revisitation narratives attempt to resolve this tension by inviting us to mourn the mass death of our potential mentors, uncles, johns, fathers, and lovers."

Identifying mourning as the narrative tactic of these nostalgic productions, Keeler advises also "seeking out these ideas and figures that have been at the edge of the frame," a tactic central to preparing for an investigation of Kelly's work. Keeler prompts, "But what if we didn't stop at mourning the dead? What if we sought out their ghosts, not to banish but to follow?" Keeler identifies the central tensions in "Other Balms, Other Gileads": "Kelly's protagonist flickers between presence and absence, between attending to her needs and dissociating from them. . . . The ecstasy of orgasm and the ecstasy of the pharmacological high collide in Kelly's story." Keeler positions the narrator as identifying "with the undead and the unhuman, with the unending practice of pleasing the body that eclipses the necessity of living in one. She abandons this expectation of living (or dying) to instead take up haunting, which isn't altogether tragic, just an alternative way of asserting her impossible existence. **She** is the ghost we must follow." Keeler reads the story as a spooky example of "monster politics," a response to "the trope of both transwomen and HIV-positive people as tragic, predatory monsters out to kill the innocent. Kelly reworks the monster-queer into a figure still predatory, but out to terrorize the very much guilty system that manages the living, the dying, and the dead": "This mode of monstrosity feels most explicit when Kelly's protagonist un-tragically calls her body 'Biohazard-ous.' In a good way, as a deterrent against unwanted sexual advances. But also as a profoundly resistant sense of queer, HIV-positive embodiment. Resistant to what, though? Cissexism? Heteropatriarchy? The Human Rights Campaign (HRC)? . . . Just as Godzilla haunts Japan as a specter of nuclear violence, the bio-hazardous queer body haunts New York City as a specter of AIDS in epidemic time." Keeler thus presents Kelly's fiction as offering "a demand for more from an AIDS Crisis Revisitation than questions of life and death: questions of embodi-ment, of pleasure, of technology, and of power." In returning to Kelly's work today—as her own ghost now also haunts us—we can think through the care she provided for her chosen family, lovers, Tumblr followers, and roommates and the "tiny acts of love" she shared with strangers in welfare office waiting rooms. As Keeler identifies, this body of work urges us to "demand for more" from all the systems that failed to adequately care for Bryn.

I Can Feel Better

In this section, I close read contemporary trans literature to trace the influence of early HIV kinships on queer and trans body self-determination in the pre-sent. Kelly's narratives of family and HIV bridge current trans fiction with the early HIV archive. While not all contemporary trans writing addresses HIV directly, the influence of early HIV activism on contemporary trans writing is significant for younger generations who continue to rescript long-standing bio-medical cultural narratives about queerness and disability. This ongoing move-ment for sexual and gender self-determination can be linked back to the early HIV archive through work like Kelly's that refuses body shame for being dis-abled and trans and for living with HIV. While Kelly's narratives of domestic care trouble idyllic visions of queer family, and Sur and Schulman address break-downs in biological kinships, Plett's short stories of parents reacting to their trans children offer additional narrative possibilities for representing not only family violence but also acceptance and care. Plett's 2014 publication *A Safe Girl to Love* presents a collection of short stories, each told from the perspective of a different trans woman. Plett's work is especially compelling as a reflection of trans women's familial experiences in that each young narrator within the col-lection depicts vastly different dynamics with her parents. In "Not Bleak," the volume's longest story, Carla discusses her difficulties with her mother. While Schulman's narrators lack this opportunity to reconcile with estranged parents, Carla describes the persistent pain of trying to rebuild a relationship after initial rejection. She brings the reader up to speed on her family drama in an insider testimonial tone reminiscent of Schulman's David. We learn that Carla's mother began speaking with her daughter again only after Carla nearly died from drinking two bottles of whisky. Carla confesses,

> I still don't really feel like I can trust her. There was a period in my life, right after we started talking again, when I tried really hard. And I told everyone my mom and I had reunited and it was all magical and amazing—the whole thing was kinda 21st-century *Lifetime* movie ready, right? But it still eats at me. I hate it. Like, how can it be love if it takes a close shave with death to see your daughter as a person? I don't see how that's love. I know that's a snarly thing to say, I know I should just move on. I feel so petty for not getting over it, but I don't know how to not hurt about that. I don't. I don't want to be all magically close and loving with my mom again. I just want to forgive her and stop hurting, I want to be calm and forgive, but I can't, I still hurt about it, I can't, I can't, I don't know how. (156–57)

This highly conversational passage is peppered with informal appeals to the listener, aural repetitions for emphasis, rhetorical questions, and even an admission that these words are snarly "to *say*" (emphasis mine). This dialogue format is noteworthy in that its distinct speech-like qualities present a paradox for the reader to ponder: this conversational passage exists in the text only for the reader's benefit and not as fodder for actual oral communication with Zeke, the young trans woman whose intimate disclosure about her own relationship to her grandfather prompts Carla's (internal) monologue.

Though Carla seems to be disclosing information, her internal narrative structure points to—through representing instances of parental cruelty—how difficult it is to truly *talk* about it. Aloud to Zeke in this moment, all Carla replies is, "That actually makes a lot of sense" (157). The narrative then presents Zeke's curt response of "Thanks" (157), at which point the impact of Carla's disclosure is interrupted via the plot when she checks a text message from her boyfriend. This pattern of cycling around parental trauma, as it subsides and later reemerges throughout the story, presents readers with a representation of familial abandonment that builds on Schulman's narrative model of showing how the experience of familial rejections cannot be ignored. Unlike Schulman's David, who spells out this process overtly for his reader, Carla sets up the persistence of familial abandonment as that which must be actively pieced together by her reader using information given about how Carla's family dynamics affect her ability to connect to other characters including Zeke. The narrative thus complicates the potential of trans chosen family to stand in for biological caregiving, as biological family rejection can increase the challenge of sustaining outside emotional connections. Plett's narrative structure, where parental trauma is buried but continually resurfaces, conveys the inassimilable nature of parental abandonment as a social-cum-personal problem. "It's shitty, but sometimes I wish my parents never talked to me again" (176), concedes Carla at the story's end:

> Sometimes I'm not glad my mom and I have a relationship. It would be less confusing. Like when I call her and ask what's happening for my dad's birthday and she says well we're free the day before. A friend once said it's hard, letting that stuff go. I can't ever *imagine* letting it go. I wish someone could teach me how. I really do. I wish I knew if they would still be outright ignoring me today if I hadn't years ago started into a second bottle of whisky. But the question's unanswerable. Not unlike the question, I guess, of how much I really wanted to die. (177)

Thus while Plett's narrative initially seems less overtly centered around familial rejection than Schulman's, it ultimately reveals the centrality of family care; seemingly minor infractions involving birthdays and communication breaches are connected to the physical suffering that results from parental rejection. While Schulman's narrator directly articulates this conundrum for the reader, Carla presents information more tentatively, thus requiring the reader's collaboration in identifying the internal effects of family trouble as a process that is not always self-evident until it becomes illuminated through the narrative process. The disability narrative here includes representations of navigating mental health by grappling with the links between parental rejection and suicidal feelings. The difficulty of even acknowledging the effects of family harm become written into the story itself. Plett's trans narrative tactics concede the effects of familial harm while still paying tribute to trans women's resilience. In the end, Plett presents the irreconcilable conundrum of parental abandonment alongside a strategy through which Carla affirms her own tenacity, as the last lines of the story affirm: "And I feel better. I can feel better" (177).

Although Plett and Schulman both represent the effects of parental rejection, Plett's narratives also investigate what is possible when biological families are able to provide queer and trans kin with care. Carla's narrative of parental abandonment is one likely familiar to readers via tropes of lesbian fiction dating back to those of Schulman, but the characters in this volume's other stories experience parental reactions to their trans-ness in a large assortment of previously un- (or at least under-)represented ways. The expansive range of family configurations stitched together through the various chapters of Plett's collection mirrors *A Safe Girl to Love*'s extensive offering of geographic settings, character types, and transfeminine gender expressions. Reading Schulman's 1990s fiction in dialogue with the recent work of Plett represents not only generational differences but also intergenerational lineages of interrogating the capacity of family in providing access to care.

Plett's fiction therefore expands the queer narrative possibilities offered by Schulman's by providing a variety of strategies for representing not only parental cruelty but also parental support. Schulman represents surviving HIV as interconnected to surviving parental rejection, and Plett extends on this queer lineage by considering how biological family can correspondingly bolster queer resilience. Although HIV is not an overt theme within the family dramas of the earlier stories, Plett's penultimate story, "Winning," draws on histories of HIV activism to offer yet another set of narrative possibilities for representing trans families and disability. This story introduces us to Zoe and to her mother Sandy, who we come to learn is also trans. Zoe's mother's (albeit temporary) abandonment of her daughter upon Zoe's coming out as trans is complicated; Sandy's emotional response to Zoe's disclosure stems not from a lack of understanding but from the experiential fears that overcome Sandy regarding her daughter's safety. Though attributed to her own trauma and not ignorance, Sandy's fears nevertheless inhibit her from actually supporting Zoe through a time when parental love is most critical. The later reconciliation between mother and daughter that structures this narrative presents an arresting moment of intimacy between the two women at Zoe's small-town childhood home:

> Zoe was finishing cleaning the garage when Sandy walked up to Zoe from behind and hugged her and burrowed her head into Zoe's neck. Then Sandy said, I love that you're my daughter, and both of them shook and cried a little in the most delicious, healthy, loving of ways, the way that only mothers and daughters can. In a way that really, in a sense, Zoe had wanted to touch her mother for twenty-four years. They stood in the garage, cold, holding each other for a long time. She thought of Sandy's parents, estranged since before Sandy had even left home, and wondered fleetingly if it was possible to love so fully, as Sandy had, unless you had been cut off at some point from that love yourself. (201)

This reconciliatory moment provides a false climax to the story. The intensity of this exchange is again diffused by the narrative through the non sequitur sending of a text message. While the contents of this text shift our focus away from the mother-daughter relationship and onto a seemingly unconnected thread of the plot, in the end this new plotline becomes an indication of the combination of love and abandonment experienced between the pair. Plett's narrative strategies extend on Schulman's earlier representations of parental abandonment as a disappearing but always reemerging symptom whose reverberating effects can again be traced through this ongoing process of queer and trans storytelling. Throughout the story cycle, Plett's writing style reveals itself as less straightforward and more conflicted as the unresolved tensions from each individual story resurface across the larger body of work. The implicit connections between mental health, resilience, disability, and familial care become more apparent although not more obvious throughout the collection, linking kinship to gender self-determination.

The representation of family trouble in Plett's fiction can be traced back to early HIV narratives that document this queer process of surviving family break-downs. There is, however, a significant narrative shift between the overt discussion of familial abandonment in novels like Schulman's and the underhanded storytelling strategies leveraged by Plett. Plett offers her readers a tempting simplicity and a narrative of familial reconciliation that again is later undercut. This pure rendering of motherly love from Sandy to Zoe characterizes the deceptively straightforward structure of not just "Winning" but the stories throughout *A Safe Girl to Love*. While it is enticing to grasp onto this offering of uncomplicated love between mother and daughter in this tender narrative moment, motherly care is never provided without accompanying harms. In spite of this gesture of armistice, Sandy later initiates an argument in the car on the way to the shopping mall. Sandy chastises Zoe's lack of inhibition about being trans together in public space: "Zoe, you can't be so cavalier. You can't" (209). Sandy's warning that her daughter "can't just sail through the world all charmed and oblivious anymore" (209) leaves Zoe "feeling tiny" (209). The conversation escalates and Sandy exclaims, "I'm serious . . . they'll find out you used to be a man!" (209). Zoe retorts, "I was never a *fucking man*, okay?" at which point Sandy adopts a tone of incredulousness and exclaims, "Ohhhh my *God! You* think you just stopped being my son, don't you? . . . Do you think that's how it works?! Do you think you went to a fucking wizard?!" (210). Sandy's differing gender analysis from Zoe's, we learn, is inseparable from her own generational experience of trauma from being outed and facing corresponding violence. In contrast to the maxim that there is safety in numbers, Sandy becomes "oddly flustered" (209) in attempting to convey to Zoe that "you tend to get into more trouble in groups" (209). Sandy's fear that being near her daughter will not protect but rather endanger her is conveyed through Plett's use of straightforward prose. Plett's under-stated language renders the tension placed on individual families attempting to mediate larger systems of violence.

Plett's storytelling strategies also capture the intricacies of the family as both supporting and undermining sexual and gender self-determination. Plett's contemporary trans fiction and Schulman's early HIV narratives can be read as interconnected in representing how biological kinships can enforce complacency or encourage disruption to body norms. Following Sandy's warning en route to the shopping mall, the pair is approached by a man who stops them to comment to Sandy, "Ma'am, if you don't mind me saying so, you have a beautiful daughter" (210). This trite expression of adoration for the women together creates an unsettling sense of discomfort for the reader as it both undercuts the mother's prior warnings and confirms the ongoing presence of nonconsensual interactions characteristic of public space. The stark contrast between Sandy's fears of discovery and this man's uninvited compliment creates an unease that is spotlighted by Zoe's reflection on passing: "She'd waited 'til she was ten months on hormones to go full-time, and she had never heard an unkind word in her direction about it. Not one episode of street harassment or threat. Of the trans variety, anyway. . . . She was lucky, she knew it; none of her friends back in New York (like Julia, fuck . . .) could say that. But she'd more or less passed from the moment she wanted to" (210). Zoe needs her mother not only to support her being trans but also to support her facing gender-based violence both personally and within her community. In addressing these caregiving needs via the narrative, Plett represents the difficult mix of encouragement and love, rejection and harm, that parents provide. This story captures the deep admiration Zoe holds for her mother in spite of conflicting feelings of pain. This fraught yet productive yearning for reconnection with parents extends on Schulman's narrative project of presenting familial abandonment as inescapable and insidious, a process depicted in Schulman's 2007 HIV novel *The Child* as something that feels like being "hit on the head with a hammer every day" (107), like "suffering daily" (107), "like trying to reconcile with a battering ram" (107). In both Plett and Schulman's work, the desire to "outrun" (Schulman, *The Child* 107) these tensions between love and pain only moves these heroines in the direction of confronting them, a paradox brought into relief within this story by the processes of narrating HIV.

This narrative influence of early HIV activism for younger generations of trans women is not addressed overtly until a moment in "Winning" where Zoe recalls the openness with which Sandy teaches her about sexuality and sex. Plett ultimately represents familial care between mother and daughter through this intergenerational transmission of HIV narratives. "Winning" illustrates mother-daughter dynamics in relation to the experience of Sandy's surviving the early years of the AIDS crisis and of imparting that experience to a second generation. Zoe recounts with fondness her first sex talk from her mother. She values how Sandy sat her down when she was "really young, before puberty" (197) to tell her that learning about safer sex *"gives you freedom, you can't imagine, the happiness and freedom. . . . It's something I want you to look forward to. I want this to be a good and healthy part of your life"* (198). Upon Zoe's recollection of this critical moment, we learn that "Zoe really admired that, especially when she found out about all of Sandy's friends who'd died during what she'd only refer to as the plague. Zoe had remembered a few of them, from when she was a kid. But only faintly, and only a few" (198). Zoe is unable to connect with her mother to share these reflections on friends lost to "the plague," much as they also cannot come together for Sandy to pass down narratives of trans survival or of the daily violence Zoe witnesses in her community. In this narrative rift between them, the prose subtly indicates how these experiences of AIDS and loss can be transmitted but never wholly understood across generational lines. Plett's fiction not only reveals such intergenerational disconnections but is itself a process of grappling with ongoing cultural strategies for representing HIV. Plett situates HIV not as the focus of the plot but as a critical narrative component alongside representations of intergenerational trans family trauma. In bringing early AIDS losses into contemporary representation, *A Safe Girl to Love* narrates families as multifaceted sites of rejection and shame, but also resilience and care. Though it does not always discuss HIV directly, Plett's work extends early HIV narratives to offer models of trans caregiving for gender self-determination into the present.

PIGGING OUT ON PASSOVER

To connect Plett's contemporary family narratives back to the early HIV archives, this final section undertakes a reading of disability kinship in the writing of De La Cruz. These archives of creating chosen family in response to HIV narrate disability as opportunity for interdependence and body self-determination. De La Cruz, who died of AIDS in 1991 at the age of thirty-seven, held leadership positions within sex work and HIV movements (see fig. 3.2). Already an organizer with Prostitutes of New York (PONY), De La Cruz joined preexisting communities of gay men and lesbians who coalesced to form grassroots HIV caregiving initiatives including the Gay Men's Health Crisis (GMHC) and People with AIDS Coalition (PWAC). De La Cruz's work is preserved through the careful archiving of these organizations' media including a range of once-mailed-out community newsletters, VHS videotapes of oral history interviews, and out-of-print magazines and books.

In these literary archives of her contributions, De La Cruz narrates HIV family formations as critical to her own survival. She advocates for kinships that bring together women living with HIV as they engage in medical self-advocacy. De La Cruz revisits her feelings of loneliness in the 1980s, prior to discovering one of the only existing support groups for women living with HIV. She recalls, "I felt like I was the only woman in the world with AIDS. . . . All of a sudden I discovered other women with the virus. There were black women, white women, Latinas, rich women, and poor women. There were addicts and transfusion women. They were mothers and sisters and lovers and daughters and grandmothers. Some were militant lesbians and others were Republicans (imagine that! Even Republicans get AIDS)" (134). Without diminishing the value of resources offered by gay male communities, De La Cruz asserts the need for women living with HIV to receive support that is gender specific (Singleton 51). In her AIDS Activist Project oral history interview, community leader and activist with AIDS ACTION NOW! (AAN) Darien Taylor similarly discusses the process of starting Voices of Positive Women, a Toronto-based organization to break isolation for women living with HIV. Taylor recalls living with HIV in Ontario in the 1980s: "It took me a long time to meet another HIV-positive woman; like, a couple of years before I met another woman with HIV." She remembers moving to Toronto and finding the AIDS Committee of Toronto but coming to

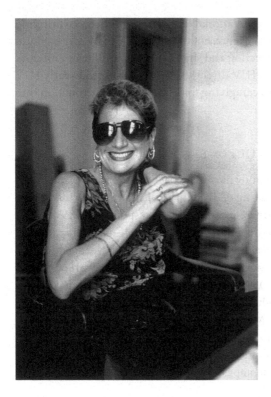

Figure 3.2. Iris De La Cruz: "I had a good time getting this disease and I'm going to have a good time dealing with it." Courtesy of Iris House.

realize that "there were no HIV-positive women around," as she details the work of creating networks for women living with HIV to come together. Taylor acknowledges the caregiving labor that happens invisibly in bringing women together to address gender-based violence and break isolation. In a GMHC Oral History interview that remains on a VHS tape in the New York Public Library (NYPL) archive, De La Cruz, like Taylor, recounts first coming into a community of women living with HIV: "I would take the subway and walk around thinking I had this giant 'A' that flashed on my forehead and everyone that looked at me could tell I had AIDS. I would look at families and lovers together and think that these are options that are no longer open to me (not anymore). I would get real depressed, seeing happy people, and I wasn't the only one that felt like that." Through attending and later leading some of the first-ever women's HIV support groups, De La Cruz narrates the impact of community care. She shares, "I started going to women's group and this sounds real cliché but I learned self-empowerment—I learned that I was responsible for my own health or my own lack of health and didn't need to worship at the altar of the AMA [American Medical Association], my doctor didn't have all the answers." De La Cruz presents gender self-determination as a community-driven form of care:

Women have to be in control of their own treatment, their own health care, because . . . if women don't act on their own, it won't get done, if you're going to sit there and wait for this magic pill that's going to make everything all right, it's not going to happen. You have to do it. And it's hard work, but now at least there is support. And there has to be some unity. . . . You can't go about taking care of this on your own. And there are a lot more women who are either undiagnosed or who they're in a closet about this . . . and they need to get together, just like they did in the late 60s early 70s in the women's health care movement they need to do it with this.

De La Cruz's caregiving work connects women living with HIV to one another and to histories of feminist medical activism through her in-person support groups and through the distribution of her narratives in community newsletters and grassroots publications. Not only did De La Cruz's work influence how her readers understood their own relationships to HIV in the 1980s and early 1990s, but her archival records can also continue to influence how we imagine disability kinships today.

Through her narratives of forming HIV kinships, De La Cruz turns the narrative scrutiny away from the person living with HIV and onto medical providers: "They did all kinds of testosterone studies—that was the first thing, god forbid that guys can't get hard-ons—they'll look at that from morning to night. I didn't menstruate for the first year of this virus and I would ask doctors and they would say, 'I don't know why.' Well, why don't you know why? If you don't know why, find out why!" Using narrative to offset the unidirectional flow of authority between doctor and patient, De La Cruz's writing models a communal process of holding practitioners responsible for eliminating gender disparities in treatment and in widening access to care. Her archives offer an ongoing sex-positive, harm reduction narrative model for body self-determination. She writes that "women—low risk people, and transfusion people— . . . would have to start off every group explaining they were low risk or they got it through a transfusion." De La Cruz recalls, "It got to the point where I said, 'this isn't the issue in this group, it might be your issue, the thing is, how are you dealing with the virus? I don't care if you fucked the Green Bay Packers. How are you dealing with this virus?" In "dealing with this virus" alongside her readership of women living with HIV, De La Cruz models the historical and ongoing creation of queer and trans chosen families as response to disability.

Although De La Cruz identifies as cisgender and straight, her queer HIV kinships include her lesbian daughter, her "AIDS militant" Jewish mother, and the gay men and lesbians who become family via acts of care. Her writing expands conceptions of family by addressing those readers estranged from their own families of origin to remind them that "they were not alone and support was available to them." In "The Great Sero-Positive Seder: Or, Pigging Out on Passover," published in the July 1990 edition of the PWAC's newsletter *Newsline*, De La Cruz narrates HIV as motivation for breaking isolation:

> My mother has started a sort of tradition. She started making Passover Seders for people dealing with HIV. This started out a couple of years ago, after I was released from the hospital with an AIDS diagnosis. It was only supposed to be a one-shot deal because I was supposed to die, but it has since evolved into an annual event. Since I spent all my time perfecting my Camille death bed scene, I had no time to make any new friends (and my old friends, I didn't want to see my old friends.) So my mom put up a sign at GMHC for PWAs who wanted a home cooked meal.

De La Cruz reframes disability as forming caregiving communities that blend biological and chosen family. Her writing style combines campy sarcasm with candid sincerity to relay how she too would have remained isolated had it not been for her mother. Recognizing the barriers to finding community, De La Cruz depicts her own reluctance to participate in Passover: "I wasn't too overjoyed about that since I wasn't all that thrilled about eating at that point. And . . . having strangers in the house would also mean I would have to be civil, which was a drag. Your family *knows* just how bitchy you can be. I looked forward to this in much the same way as I'd look forward to dining on crushed glass." In creating rapport with her readers, De La Cruz indulges in some self-deprecation (Jewish humor) to represent the intricacies of coping with terminal illness and isolation. This tactic of surviving through humor is also recalled by Joy Episalla in an *ACT Up Oral History Project* interview where she remembers her friend James Baggett: "he was just such a sweet guy—just lovely. Very, very funny. He had a great sense of humor. He'd say things to me—when we'd be at an ACT UP demonstration and they'd be saying, 'ACT UP, Fight Back, Fight AIDS!'—he'd be whispering in my ear, 'ACT UP, Fried Eggs!'" (22). De La Cruz likewise positions survival as connected to her capacity for sharing laughter communally, in caring for others who are also "dealing with HIV." Using narrative to reach out to a readership of "true miracles who can laugh at . . . themselves," De La Cruz links caregiving to the playfulness of storytelling. She declares for her readers that "we will survive on our snickering."

In narrating HIV caregiving as a powerful site for "snickering," De La Cruz's Passover story uses humor to reframe disability as generating queer kinships. De La Cruz details the vulnerabilities and intimacies of exchanging care through the process of collective laughter. Deborah Gould analyzes this use of humor by ACT UP as a strategy for coping with violence and mass deaths from AIDS in the 1980s and 1990s, of using camp and style to continue to survive and to make activism sustainable and fun (197). De La Cruz's *Newsline* column, "Kool-AIDS (With Ice)," uses camp narratives to support social and sexual networks through this act of writing and reading. Today this includes the original readers of the *Newsline*, but even those of us generations later who never had a chance to meet De La Cruz can still be moved by the pleasure she took in forming HIV communities. De La Cruz, for instance, used her writing to publicize the PWAC's upcoming events, including "our infamous HIV dance," "a chance to get dressed up and act slutty!" De La Cruz muses,

> I haven't been out dancing in so long . . . are they still doing the frug? So since I haven't gotten my hip-hop down pat, I guess I'll have to make up my own steps. The first one is that old standard, the I.V. pole waltz. This is done using an I.V. pole as a partner. If you still have a line hooked up, that's even better since it shows intimacy and a common bond between you and your partner. There is nothing as graceful as seeing this done in perfect unison and not like me who ran into people (usually nurses) and ended up caroming the pole off the walls trying to navigate turns. Then we have the neuropathy jerk. This is done with the arms or legs held (or both) held stiff. These people have been known to do a great robot too. Real romantic is the tuberculosis tango. This is where both partners dance to a regular tango up to the minute where they dip and then they both break down into wild hacking fits of coughing. Preferably in one another's face. This shows commitment and longing. Especially for oxygen. If performed right, it will bring tears to the eyes.

De La Cruz's humor reframes the disabled body as a site of pleasure and laughter. Playing on the body's various "longings," De La Cruz connects sexual desire to other forms of survival and bodily functions. By writing about these processes for a community of readers living with HIV, De La Cruz creates excitement for the upcoming dance while simultaneously building an archive of its historical existence. In caring for this archive, we might also find joy in dancing in hospital rooms and in imagining ourselves as members of her readership, even decades later as her words take on new meanings for queer and trans body self-determination.

De La Cruz's campy narrative tactics also reflect the queer early HIV activist aesthetics of this period. For instance, filmmaker John Goss's 1989 production, *Stiff Sheets*, provides a "Fabulous Fascist Fashion Show" to protest health-care atrocities made apparent by HIV. Staged in front of LA County/USC Medical Hospital as part of a larger demonstration by ACT UP/LA, the show features drag queens sporting fashions like knee-length pink triangle dresses and full-body "Band Aids!" which the campy master of ceremonies reminds us are "the official solution to the AIDS epidemic." A group of models strut down the runway in jogging suits, as the MC annotates, "Night Sweats: more than a fashion, it's a condition, more than a style, it's a symptom." The announcer marvels that "these Sweats attract little or no attention at all. It took 8 years of federal inaction to perfect this outfit, and it will last a lifetime." The show concludes with a finale of "homophobes on parade," where the runway models don the masks of celebrities from Buckley to Reagan. De La Cruz uses this queer humor to narrate HIV as a site of pleasure through which different bodies can connect toward fighting medical injustice and building interdependence (Wendell 145; Withers, *Disability* 109). In spite of De La Cruz's initial hesitations about Passover, she writes, "our guests came, unknown and unwanted (by me), and wonder of wonders, I had a good time." She continues, in camp style, to re-center the role of domestic labor within family dynamics: "What made it even better, was the fact that I was still pretty sick, so I got out of doing dishes." In calling attention to the undesirability of domestic chores, De La Cruz effectively makes apparent the labor of planning, cooking, and cleaning that remains an essential though often invisible component of bringing people together. De La Cruz reveals the outcome of her mother's labor in facilitating a community Passover: "What ended up happening was we all became friends and an annual tradition was born. I guess nobody thought I would ever live this long. Certainly not me." Because the Passover ritual always concludes by looking forward to the next year's event, De La Cruz's writing envisions community through sustained HIV connections over time.

Unburying these HIV narratives across time reanimates the past as informing new types of disability kinships in the present. As we read these archives now, our understandings of queer and trans chosen family can be shaped by these narratives of early HIV caregiving. Through her writing, De La Cruz links her own physical survival with the formation of HIV family. She shares her experience of disability as interconnected to the communities disability creates: "This past Passover found me still alive. And healthy enough to do dishes. . . . And then there was the question of who to invite. I had a lot more friends this year than I did when I was diagnosed. . . . The guys that came before were also present this year, along with the assorted perverts that comprise my family and friends." Such retellings of the Passover of "assorted perverts" presents a queer kinship model that blends biological and chosen family, what Tim Dean theorizes as "the various ways that people could become related to each other by blood without involving heterosexuality" (90). The Passover Seder—traditionally understood as an intimate participatory ritual open to strangers and wanderers from outside of one's own community—represents the widening of who might be included around the table as family (Levine 258). Thus in opposition to stigmatizing narratives that frame disability as an individual, biomedical problem to be cured (McRuer, *Crip* 231; Clare, *Brilliant* 183), HIV caregiving narratives expand notions of family toward increasing accessibility and support. De La Cruz includes her readers in this collective process, addressing us directly in concluding, "I guess if I stay alive, we'll have to do this every year. So listen up, you guys, on our twentieth anniversary, we're gonna *really* kick it!! Thank mom." This readership inclusion in kinship formation continues even decades later: as De La Cruz's readers—even after her own death—we are still addressed by her narrative call as active members of her PWA Passover guest list. Taking this literature out of its temporal context allows De La Cruz and her legacy to reverberate posthumously, closing the gap in time between the early years of HIV and current disability activism.

The chosen families formed through these narratives can therefore connect generations who lived through the early years of HIV to younger queer and trans readers hoping to learn about these histories. De La Cruz creates a dialogue about her own care needs that includes her readers in her process of self-advocacy. The role of her readership is always a significant component of De La Cruz's narrative process, as her direct address to readers forms a bridge between understanding disability as an individual versus social experience. The genre of the public narrative builds connections between people living with HIV and people experiencing similar obstacles to receiving gender-specific care. De La Cruz's narratives thereby hold the potential to connect early HIV activism with a variety of other medical access barriers to body self-determination that queer and trans people continue to form families and caregiving networks in order to better navigate.

While Schulman's novels illustrate the caregiving gaps that arise when biological family fails, and Plett's short stories extend on these failures to illustrate what happens when biological family is supportive, De La Cruz's autobiographical reflections blend biological and chosen family to address the limits and possibilities of both models by combining them in unlikely places like the hospital. This melding of biological and chosen family networks reframes how we form family in response to our bodies' pleasures, limitations, and collaborations, none of which need to be understood as mutually exclusive. Throughout her writing, De La Cruz foregrounds her mother's instrumental role in helping her navigate medical discrimination. De La Cruz remembers her hospitalization for advanced tuberculosis, recalling how "the hospital staff tried doing things at their convenience. They were messing with the wrong one." De La Cruz recalls that while she was in the hospital, "food was the last thing on my mind. So my mother came up armed with corned beef and ice cream and sat there by my bed until I consented to take a bite." Taking the dismal situation of feeling too ill to eat and turning it into a humorous moment, De La Cruz performs her own body's care needs in a lighthearted and public way to relay for her readers the importance of family support. De La Cruz jokes, "Jewish mothers, by law, must take a course in 'nudgery.' . . . my mother could be an instructor [. . . she] bugged me into walking, and, when I was released, into getting out of the house. Needless to say, I'm well enough now to the point where she feels she can bug me about house work." De La Cruz attributes her mother's care to her surviving what was diagnosed as a terminal stay in the hospital. De La Cruz also commends her mother for creating the PWA Passover Seders and for helping to reunite other people living with HIV with their own estranged parents. In narrating this disability kinship,

De La Cruz frames caregiving as a process of both creating chosen family and reinforcing links between biological family members. De La Cruz narrates how her activist work is fueled not only by anger but by the support of her mother and by her love for her lesbian daughter: "My child is now 19 and we're very close. The legacy I want to leave her is for her to remember her mama was a survivor. She survived drugs and she survived her own worst enemy, which was herself. And she taught others survival. She may or may not have survived AIDS, but she kicked ass while she was here" (134). De La Cruz's kinship models inspire a shift away from individual biomedical narratives about disability, creating gender self-determination through her collective narratives of laughing together and living with HIV. She offers contemporary readers this legacy of building queer and trans kinships through the intimacies, humor, and even the failures of care: "I know that [the virus is] there, but I can live with it. This is what I try to teach the people that come to my groups. You can live with this. If you survive drugs and all the bullshit, all the discrimination, you can survive AIDS. Or at least while you're alive you can live."

The fiction and autobiographical writing surveyed throughout this chapter narrates a contradictory combination of anger and love, desire and care that family creates. While De La Cruz and Plett present narratives of chosen family as including biological kin, Schulman and Kelly narrate the harms that arise from families failing to care for disability and difference. These narratives thus understand parental love as potentially bolstering gender self-determination but also as necessitating the formation of broader supports for when family caregiving fails. Reading these narratives offers younger generations models of collective laughter and of bringing people together to support queer and trans survival. Chapter 4 will further consider the representation of disability kinships in the HIV caregiving narratives of Rebecca Brown. Brown's work reframes HIV as motivating queer intimacies that support reciprocal care. However, *The Gifts of the Body* curiously removes details of the narrator's personal life from her own autobiographically based narrative. Chapter 4 reads Brown's narrative withholding as a literary strategy for reframing care as a desire-driven, mutual process. As this chapter has shown, narratives of HIV caregiving can continue to expand ongoing definitions of disability as well as narrative representations of chosen family that queer and trans kinds of caregiving create.

CHAPTER 4

The Gift of Dykes

NAMING DESIRE IN REBECCA BROWN'S
NARRATIVES OF CARE

Rebecca Brown's HIV narratives reframe disability as a site of mutual desire through the exchange of care. Extending on the archives of HIV–chosen family in chapters 1 to 3, Brown's literary models of disability kinship offer representations of early HIV caregiving toward creating interconnectivity. Unlike Brown's 1993 short story "A Good Man," which characterizes its lesbian narrator through her familial kinship with her gay best friend, *The Gifts of the Body*, published only one year later, excludes nearly all information about the unnamed narrator's personal life. Such omissions raise questions about how and why this narrator's queerness, like her identity more broadly, remains unnamed. Like family trauma in the fiction of Sarah Schulman and Casey Plett, the (likely autobiographically based) narrator in *The Gifts of the Body* surfaces and disappears, creating slippages between genders and sexualities, caregivers and recipients, able-bodiedness and disability. The openness of Brown's narrative depicts caregiving as a potentially reciprocal process that breaks down the distinction between giving and receiving support. The narrator's elusiveness also strategically renders how caregiving can often become unbalanced, unnamed, and a site of emotional withdrawal, mirroring the larger withholding patterns central to the narrative itself. Close-reading these gaps attends not only to what Brown depicts but also to what she conceals, offering a complex narrative of mutual care that connects early HIV narratives to queer and trans disability representations in the present.

In this chapter, I take up an investigation of queer representation in Brown's literature to imagine how the kinds of kinships formed through HIV caregiving continue to influence sexual and gender self-determination. Interestingly, the queer intimacies represented by Brown are not always named as such, complicating definitions of what might constitute sexual or gendered aspects of exchanging care. I read queerness within Brown's fiction as offering a model of care that brings bodies together in a potentially mutual exchange in spite of the ways care provision can also cause emotional or physical distance between care-giver and recipient, narrator and reader. The structure of this chapter begins by looking at queer caregiving relationships in "A Good Man" in order to consider how practices of naming, withholding, and exchange function within the full-length *Gifts*. In reading these texts together, I argue that queer gender expression and queer sexual desire are central to the formation of HIV caregiving kinships, in spite of—and even because of—the fact that *Gifts'* narrator's queerness is never named as such. *Gifts* is significant as a work of fiction because it represented queer-ness and HIV for a mainstream audience to cultural and critical acclaim during the early years of HIV via its portrayal of women's care work. Reading Brown's HIV literature remains influential in the present, as taking these narratives back up offers the opportunity to understand how early queer representations of HIV and care continue to shape fluid queer and trans genders and sexualities.

Through literary representations of caregivers and care recipients coming together to mutually exchange needs, names, and even body fluids, *Gifts* uses these narrative withholding strategies to uncover the power dynamics of care. Brown's tactics of naming (and not naming) and her coded depictions of her nar-rator's sexuality reframes HIV caregiving as fluid and as reciprocally driven by queer sexual desire and mutual exchange. Brown's work is important as litera-ture because the seemingly straightforward genre in which she writes about HIV offers complex and experimental models for depicting (and withholding) care. Like Brown's larger corpus of realist/experimental lesbian fiction and memoir, her HIV narratives reframe bodily differences, limits, and pain as generative rather than as something to be assimilated into gender or sexual norms. Read-ing Brown's early HIV literary narratives in the present grapples with the kinds of self-erasure required to give and to narrate care. The gap she creates between narrator and reader actually opens a narrative space for younger generations to connect early HIV caregiving to the challenges and pleasures of ongoing queer and trans disability kinships. Because Brown plays with the reader's expectations by undercutting the reliability and straightforwardness of the narrator's obser-vations, the reader becomes witness to the exchanges of desire that transpire through care. While *Gifts* initially appears to establish a model of caregiving that disappears care providers in favor of care recipients, a closer reading actually offers a narrative model of disability as generating interconnectivity through these very bodily and power differences. Revisiting these tensions connects early HIV caregiving literature to ongoing narratives that support kin who fail to con-form to body norms.

So Good with Her Hands

This section will look to "A Good Man" as a literary model of the sexual and gender-fluid kinships that form through HIV caregiving, rendering disability as a site of potentially mutual exchange. In her short story "A Good Man," Brown presents a queer tale of love and friendship, representing intimacy between our lesbian narrator and her gay best friend, Jim, through the exchange of care. The friends regard each other as members of each other's "family" (103), as Jim proclaims to the narrator at a Gay Pride rally, "Every single screaming fairy prancing down this boulevard and every last one of you pissed-off old Amazons is my family. My kith and my kin and my kind. My siblings. Your siblings" (112). These familial connections of queerness are emblematized by Jim's late lover, Scott, whose memory is revisited in photographs where he stands "holding up a Stonewall fist and grinning" (140). Linking queer kinship to queer revolution, the family becomes not the site of gender or sexual norms but support for nonconforming bodies to unite against the police. Whereas Scott's character posthumously signifies queerness-as-resistance, his death leaves Jim without an immediate family, causing Jim to become closer with the narrator as she cares for Jim during his initial period of mourning. The two are bound together by AIDS loss and by mutual acts of support. As their friendship develops, Jim repeatedly reinforces for the narrator the importance of refusing to hide or apologize for so-called sexual and gender deviance. Warning his friend of the dangers of shame and of feeling forced to "crawl back into the nearest closet" (112), Jim encourages the narrator to hold up her "sweet gorgeous sexy face" (112) and march alongside him in the streets: "Jim pranced back to me and yanked me into a chorus line where everyone, all these brave, tough pansies, these heroic, tender dykes, had their arms around each others' backs. Jim pulled me along. I felt the firmness of his chest against my shoulder" (113). With an intimacy that is not sexual but is nevertheless expressed through physical connections between queer bodies (e.g., through the very *firmness* of Jim's chest), their relationship becomes at once familial and queer, a bond that proves invaluable to the narrator's later role of caring for Jim (Califia 198; Gould 257).

Although the intimacy between the narrator and Jim is nonsexual, Jim feels compelled to involve himself in the romantic pursuits of his emotionally guarded and dateless best friend. Brown renders the pair's desire as a vicarious process, as the two consummate their own relationship through persistent attempts to bestow one another with dates. The narrator explains, "Jim still desired, despite what he'd been through with Scott, despite how his dear brotherhood was crumbling, that some of his sibling outlaws would find good love and live in that love openly" (102–3). As her "sibling outlaw," Jim is constantly cruising on the narrator's behalf, employing various strategies—from charming strangers at bars to placing personal ads in her name. At once humored and annoyed by her friend's brazen gestures, our narrator justifies this behavior as that which allows Jim to extend the family in spite of his loss of Scott: "His talk, his ploys to find someone for me, were his attempts to make the story of a good romance come true" (102). In *Rebecca Brown: Literary Subversions of Homonormalization*, Lies

Xhonneux also traces this process by which "gays and lesbians frequently perform acts of kinship that build new family arrangements which involve reciprocal obligations and which provide care, affection, and (material and emotional)
support" (160–61). "A Good Man," Xhonneux observes, represents chosen families making visible these alternatives to heterosexual, biological family norms
(*Rebecca* 161). The friendship between the narrator and Jim indeed offsets norms
for what a primary caregiving relationship might traditionally look like; "A Good
Man" represents desire, partnership, intimacy, and love outside of a sexual relationship or traditional hetero family unit.

This queer familial structure also carries over from the realm of "screaming"
and "prancing" and Pride, and into spaces of disability. The narrator, for example, labels herself as Jim's sister to gain access to hospital privileges denied to
"friends." Brown links desire and disability in the hospital when Jim points out
the sexual tension between his friend and his doctor. He repeatedly teases the
narrator with observations like, "Don't you think she's cute? I think she's cute.
Almost as cute as you are when you blush" (104–5). This act of narrating desire
in medical spaces provides a narrative contrast to the mainstream HIV media
of this period which, as Steven Kruger identifies, reflect homophobic cultural
tendencies of linking gay desire with impending death (78). Narrating HIV not
as a desexualized site of shame but as a source of queer kinship is a literary tactic that refuses to separate disability from desire (Kohnen 101). The potentially
somber hospital sequences are skillfully eroticized through Brown's carefully
crafted prose. In this moment of diagnosis, we are lured not into the typical narrative of AIDS symptoms premeditating a tragic decline but into a queer role-
play fantasy involving Jim's doctor. As Dr. Allen checks up on her patient, she
also checks his "sister" out. While the cadence and rhythm of Brown's writing
do not outwardly mark her writing as ostentatious or as sexually charged, the
pace of her prose positions us within an understated but perceptibly erotic environment. Symptoms and body parts are agreeably listed: "Dr. Allen feels Jim's
pulse, his forehead, listens to his chest. She asks him to open his mouth. She asks
him how it's going today . . . how nice it is that Jim has such nice visitors, then
tells him she'll see him later. . . . I stare out the window as hard as I can" (104).
The caregiving narrative transforms the hospital into a queer cruising zone and
a locus of lesbian desire (Hogan 3). Jim describes his doctor for the narrator's
benefit as being "so good with her hands" (104). In the presence of Jim's doctor,
the narrator experiences flirtation alongside an increasing awareness of the
severity of Jim's condition: "I turn away and stare out the window again. Sure
I'm blushing. And sure, I'm thinking about Dr. Allen. But what I'm thinking is
why, when she was looking at him, she didn't say 'you're looking good today, Jim.'
Or . . . we're gonna have to let you out of here soon, Jim, you're getting too healthy
for us" (105). By aligning the narrator's sexuality with Jim's illness, Brown creates a paradigm in which desire and disability are intertwined, reflecting what

Xhonneux identifies as moving away from narratives of cure by representing care (*Rebecca* 180). In framing the hospital as a queer space of flirtation rather than as a desexualized zone, Brown counters narratives that render disabled bodies as undeserving of or unfit for giving and receiving pleasure. In rendering Jim's sick body as a source of reciprocal care, the narrative's objective becomes not to victimize Jim but to enjoy the kinds of relationality he models for the narrator. This "shift from cure to care" (Xhonneux, *Rebecca* 180), therefore, strives not to eliminate disability but to depict it as propelling the lesbian narrator out of her own isolation while building queer intimacy between her and Jim.

This literary centering of the narrator's relationship with Jim (as opposed to with, say, Dr. Allen) further challenges the (hetero) norms of the romance narrative, as this love story between a lesbian and a gay man values queer connections that are intimate without hierarchizing the physical act of sex. CJ Chasin discusses how relationships on the asexual/ace spectrum that are not defined by sex or sexual desire are often derided or misunderstood for not conforming to heteronormative expressions of desire (176). "A Good Man" works against these cultural narratives that all primary partnerships should necessarily be sexual and that marriage is the highest form of interpersonal connection between two adults. The caregiving relationship between the narrator and Jim rescript the normative narrative progression toward the couple and marriage by offering readers a queer story of friendship (Pearl, *AIDS Literature* 148; Stepić 4). Brown's writing thus offers enviable alternatives to homonormative romance narratives that rely on marriage, racism, and class disparities to create state recognition—for some queers at the expense of others—within the public sphere (Pearl, *AIDS Literature* 145; Eng 7). Returning to the disability kinships of "A Good Man" models a narrative framework that troubles the prevalent contemporary queer longing for neoliberal family models and cultural assimilation (Pearl, *AIDS Literature* 145; Woubshet 23). Through the genre of the caregiving narrative, Brown offers younger generations models of queer family that do not rely on normativity, conformity, sex-negativity, or the state.

Through this queer intimacy between the narrator and Jim, "A Good Man" also reframes narratives of care as building reciprocity between care providers and recipients. Jim's illness, for instance, becomes the impetus for the narrator to begin dating again after a painful breakup with her girlfriend. Caring, the plot reinforces, is not a unidirectional process between the narrator and Jim but a mutual act. Jim consoles the narrator and encourages her to move past her destructive relationship. Rather than rendering caregiving as a one-sided process in which caregivers must put their own needs and desires aside, Brown constructs the relationship between the narrator and Jim as one of emotional vulnerability. Jim repeatedly expresses his desire to see his best friend find a new lover. He rallies her to "clean it up, girl. As a favor to the Ranger? As a favor to the ladies?" (109). Inspiring his caregiver to "take care" (109) of her "luscious"

(109) self, the inverted caregiving dynamic between the narrator and Jim prompts the reader to recognize the ways in which people living with HIV provide care to their caregivers through sharing knowledge about sexuality, queer family formations, emotional vulnerability, and survival (Xhonneux, *Rebecca* 179, 162; Gould 257). Rather than providing a sociological or anthropological study into how this process occurs, literature asserts this mutuality at the level of representation, thereby challenging the cultural narratives that often frame needing care as indicating chasteness, as dependency, and as causing burden. By using narrative to reframe caregiving as a sexy, reciprocal, and queer bonding process, Brown expands the possibilities for representing this mutuality of HIV caregiving, providing a literary framework for building ongoing antiassimilationist, self-determined disability kinships into the present.

Brown also models a literary strategy for shifting the narrative of concern away from the person living with HIV and onto the caregiver. Brown rescripts one-sided narratives that reduce disabled bodies to taking help from able-bodied caregivers (Wendell, *Rejected* 109). Instead, the caregiving exchange between bodies is represented as mutual, with help narrated as a dynamic process that flows in both directions. Jim sends the narrator chocolates at work to cheer her up after a painful run-in with her ex-girlfriend, making her "the talk, the envy of the office for a week" (111). As the narrator begins to provide emotional support for Jim after Scotty's death, Jim reciprocates with panache: "Jim sweet-talked my apartment manager into letting him into my tiny little studio apartment so he could leave me six—*six*—vases of flowers around my room when I turned twenty-seven. He taught me how to iron shirts" (111). As queer family, the two even spend the night together in order to provide mutual care: "I slept on his couch, the mornings after we'd both had more than either of us could handle and didn't want to be in our apartments alone" (11). Jim and the narrator's queer love reimagines relationship models for intimate partnerships by building a connection premised on reciprocating acts of support. Revising this early HIV narrative continues to locate disability as an ongoing opportunity to reimagine the scope and function of the connections that develop through the mutual exchange of care.

But I Understood

This next section moves from "A Good Man" to a reading of the HIV kinships that form in *Gifts*, even when the narrator's queerness remains unnamed as such. Unlike the showcasing of dyke/fag disability kinship in "A Good Man," Brown's *The Gifts of the Body* presents an HIV narrative that appears to withhold the queerness of its caregiver. The discrepancies between these two texts, however, actually uncover narrative strategies for representing the intimacies that can form through the vulnerabilities of care. Published the year after "A Good Man" was released, *Gifts* presents significant variations to this caregiving story beyond merely extending its length. Unlike "A Good Man," where the narrator's queer desires are fundamental, *Gifts* features a protagonist whose private life we learn essentially nothing about. Although queerness remains present in *Gifts* through its intimate portrayal of caring for gay men, its narrator reveals very little about her own sexuality or personal relationships. Another noteworthy shift between the two texts is their mode of distribution. "A Good Man" was independently published by City Lights in a volume of Brown's short stories and received little critical attention at the time of its release; Brown's full-length narrative was later released by HarperCollins to mainstream publicity and critical acclaim. The omission of the narrator's queerness in this more widely distributed revisiting of "A Good Man's" earlier themes may reflect the larger cultural trend toward coding queer and trans representation within mainstream publishing. Reading these two texts together raises questions of why *Gifts'* narrator cannot again be represented as a queer participant in her HIV communities. While the narrator of "A Good Man" provides care for her existing queer kin, *Gifts'* narrator's caregiving is now regulated through the service provision and nonprofit industrial complexes. Xhonneux reads the narrator's withholding of personal information in *Gifts* as an indication that she loses herself in the process of providing care (*Rebecca* 182). Xhonneux also argues that the narrator's self-erasure is a tactic intended to divert the narrative away from herself in order to hold more space for people living with HIV (*Rebecca* 182). Xhonneux cites Katrien De Moor's reading that the conspicuous absence of the narrator's voice is an indication of caregiving burnout (*Rebecca* 183). Reinforcing this understanding of care as causing caregivers to exceed their capacities or erase themselves, Diane M. Kimoto's work also characterizes HIV care provision as a strain on "interpersonal relations, social life, and financial status" (157). These investigations of what Kimoto labels "the burden of care" (157) fail to recognize the potential of caregiving to bolster (rather than "burden") "interpersonal relations, social life, and financial status" and (as Loree Erickson reminds us) sexual life as well (Erickson, "Revealing" 45). Citing Joan Tronto and De Moor's work, Xhonneux analyzes Brown's project of identifying the power dynamics between care providers and recipients in order to contest the devaluing of caregiving (*Rebecca* 186). Thus in opposition to confining care to a "burden" or "exceptional activity" (*Rebecca* 186), Brown's narrative reframes caregiving as essential (Xhonneux, *Rebecca* 186; Wendell, *Rejected* 151; Erickson, "Revealing" 45). As disability scholars remind us, because an able-bodied state is always temporary, interdependence and caregiving are fundamental to the human experience (Xhonneux, *Rebecca* 186; Wendell, *Rejected* 150–51). Read alongside "A Good Man," *Gifts* also represents the queer pleasures and mutualities that undercut capitalist forms of exchange through caregiving kinships. The unnamed queerness in *Gifts* can thus be decoded alongside, rather than against, those with whom the narrator exchanges care. While burnout and self-erasure are certainly possible readings here, the textual openness of *Gifts* also invites searching for information that we are *not* given about our narrator in order to complicate narratives about care. Brown's writing prompts readers to attend not only to what we are told but interestingly, to also look for those details that are withheld. In paying attention to what we do not know and why, the depiction of care in *Gifts* does not merely read as self-erasure, but these narrative gaps ultimately depict the inverse of burnout, the exchange of mutual support.

From the start, Brown's reader is denied a central piece of information, that of the narrator's name. Though first-person narrators like that of "A Good Man" can still attain intimacy with the reader without formally introducing themselves, *The Gifts of the Body*'s narrator's namelessness epitomizes her ongoing hesitancy to disclose information about herself to her reader. This namelessness also leaves open to interpretation whether this narrator is an autobiographical version of Brown herself, whether she is named "Rebecca Brown" or something else, and whether this is a work of life writing or of fiction. Compared with the casual absence of the narrator's name in "A Good Man" (though she is nicknamed by Jim), the absolute and prolonged anonymity of *Gifts*' narrator is disconcerting, precisely because her namelessness accentuates her ongoing withholding of any details connected to her personal life. The absence of the narrator's name also holds greater weight in the full-length work than in the short story because of the prominent role naming takes on regarding the secondary characters. Because naming and the use of given names throughout the text signify vulnerability both interpersonally and in terms of illness, Brown's narrator's namelessness can be identified as especially significant. Connected to Brown's conspicuous refusal to provide her narrator's name is her corresponding decision to conceal this narrator's sexual identity. This evasion of the narrator's sexuality could be connected to what Alexandra Juhasz argues is a greater erasure of lesbian sexual representations in the context of HIV: "In the media's pictured world, lesbians should not, and therefore do not, lead sexual lives. They are desexed through non-imagery" (170). It is this "non-imagery" that becomes particularly perplexing in *Gifts*, as naming practices (or lack thereof) might also participate in this representational problem. However, while the namelessness of lesbian desire is a problem to consider in the wider context of HIV representation (Roth and Fuller 2), the lack of naming lesbianism in *Gifts* does not eliminate the possibility of reading queer kinship as a structuring force throughout the text, as it is in "A Good Man." While one possible reading of *Gifts* is to regard the narrator's queerness as an absence, her sexuality can instead be interpreted as an unnamed but crucial component of the narrative that offers readers reciprocal narrative models of care.

This naming of characters and their queer desires also remains important—albeit often imperceptibly—in driving the plot. The significance of naming in

Gifts is first illustrated through the narrator's interactions with Connie, an elderly suburban client living with HIV for whom the narrator is a homecare provider. Connie's request that the narrator use her given name marks their newly established level of intimacy. This relational shift is accompanied by Connie's disclosure of her late husband's death and how she survived it. The narrator recalls that "after she told me all that, she told me to call her Connie instead of Mrs. Lindstrom. That took me a while to get used to, but I did" (20). This period of adjustment between the use of the formal "Mrs. Lindstrom" and the familiar "Connie" actually transpires instantly in the narrative, over the course of a single paragraph. As a result, the intimacies exchanged between the two women during this period also remain unnamed. Although perhaps not initially noticeable, we do not learn whatever informalities Connie extracts from our narrator to place the two on a first-name basis. This enhanced level of comfort that naming indicates is relevant to the plot development because it also permits the narrator to provide better services as a caregiver: "then after I'd called her Connie for a while, she said would I help her with her bath. That was the last thing she'd kept doing herself" (20). The vulnerability that naming signifies is what allows Connie to reveal her missing breast, which is also named as marking her body's history with cancer as well as her site of exposure to HIV. The narrator shares with her readers her observations on Connie's scar: "There was a big flat dent on half her chest, and a long white scar where they'd cut it off. The scar wasn't shiny, but it was old. They'd cut it off before they tested the blood supplies" (20). Although initially the narrator admits to us that she feels "afraid of the scar" (22), her ability to connect to Connie on an interpersonal level instills a sense of trust, allowing her to "wash the place around the scar" (22), an act of intergenerational caregiving intimacy through which the narrator's fears are negotiated. This intimacy does not merely indicate the significance of naming practices in the text; it marks a gap in disclosure by indicating how there is information that Connie receives, even though we do not.

As Connie and our narrator become increasingly familiar, the act of naming amasses increasing significance. Brown's use of names highlights a narrative discrepancy between the vulnerabilities we witness about Connie versus the absence of information we receive about the narrator. Although our narrator conceals nearly everything about her own personal life, she discloses a plethora of small but private details concerning Connie's illness. The narrator names all of Connie's children, "Diane and Ingrid and Joe" (19), and even her cat, "Miss Kitty" (19), while also enumerating in great detail her physical symptoms, such as her rapidly diminishing appetite: "She looked down at the plate. She took a deep breath, let it out, took another bite, chewed, swallowed. For the third bite she tried some egg. . . . On the fourth bite I heard her hold it in her mouth. After a few seconds she swallowed some but not all of it. Then after a few more seconds she swallowed the rest of it" (63–64). The macabre feeling established by the relaying of the minutiae of Connie's eating patterns is typical of the horror genre characteristic of Brown's earlier work. The discomfort of our voyeuristic presence mirrors the narrator's own feigned distraction during this scene: "I was still looking toward the TV, but I could hear what she was doing" (63). While the narrator names none of the figures—lovers, friends, or family members—central to her own life, she continues to demonstrate her growing bond with Connie through the act of naming kin. For example, Connie's increasing comfort with the narrator is signaled through the act of naming her husband: "she used to refer to him as her late husband, but now she just called him her husband, or John" (56). Connie in turn attempts to solicit details about her caregiver's life by asking the narrator a series of cursory questions: "She started talking. She asked me where I lived in town, in a house or an apartment, if I had pets and so on, all nice polite questions someone that age would ask" (15). While introductory questions such as these are indeed "polite," they can potentially play a complicated role for queers, as innocuous questions about one's living situation or pet ownership can easily precipitate a risky moment of disclosure related to coming out. Politeness, especially in relationships mediated by power structures such as the client/caregiver dynamic, can become quite precarious: revealing the seemingly mundane details of day-to-day life could be potentially threatening to one's employment status or could be too intimate for the initial moments of a new acquaintance.

Yet, as their relationship develops and the narrator and Connie learn more about one another's lives, the questions relayed for our benefit remain disappointingly "polite": "she asked me where I'd gone to college and what my interests were and about my family and hobbies and pets" (19). Under this potentially revealing rubric of "family," a category that could include our narrator's lover, no comment is made regarding private affairs of any sort. Although one might initially presume that the narrator hesitates to disclose information because Connie's response could be homophobic, Connie's closeness with her gay son and his partner demonstrates otherwise. Connie even laments the fraught relationship between her husband, John, their queer son, Joe, and Joe's partner, Tony (who, unlike the narrator, are all named): "'I wish he and Joe had been able to see through their differences before John died. I know they'd have come to understand and forgive each other.' Her voice shook. 'It's been very hard on Joe.' Her mouth was trembling" (159). Connie confides to the narrator, "John died of a heart attack. . . . There were things left unresolved. He hadn't seen Joe in ages. And he'd only met Tony that once" (158). While our narrator's lack of disclosure in response to Connie's intimate confession might seem to carry "politeness" to an unnecessary level, a closer examination of Brown's sparse prose proves far more telling than any information we directly receive.

Although *Gifts* certainly lacks the easily legible queerness of "A Good Man," a closer reading of this cryptic novel provides insight into how the narrator's queer gender and sexuality actually remain indirectly implied and yet highly influential throughout. Brown's decision to make queerness less overt (rather than absent) offers a different (rather than antithetical) way of narrating the impact of queer intimacies as supporting mutual care. For instance, upon learning of John's rejection of his gay son, the narrator remarks quite simply, "I hadn't known any of this before, but I understood" (158). These understated but deceptively important words, "I understood," could suggest a link between Joe's homosexuality and the narrator's own queerness, a link that could be quite apparent to Connie but not to us. In fact, the narrator's paltry self-disclosures again expose that Connie holds far more information about our narrator than is revealed to the reader. That which the narrator willfully omits could be as important as what she provides. One major set of details that Connie knows, which we do not, are the physical attributes belonging to the narrator—the contours of her face, her style of hair, her mode of dress—factors all clear to Connie but hidden from the reader. While queerness in literature is necessarily signified through linguistic description, queerness in everyday life is often also determined through a series of observable cues that "inscribe the body . . . in ways that offend the perceived sexual and embodiment norms of heterodominant culture" (Pitts 444). Such cues are readily apparent as indicators of belonging to others who also participate in queer communities, a process explained in Imogen Binnie's 2013 trans punk novel *Nevada* as "specifics" (184): "Do you want to be in a band? Do you want to have lots of weird sex, no sex, lots of weird vegan food, a haircut that reads like a secret code that identifies you as a member of a subculture to other members of that subculture?" (184). Gleaning information about queerness in literature thus requires more maneuvering on the part of the reader than a simple "secret code" haircut could readily provide in real life. In her reading of "A Good Man," Xhonneux points to the limits of reading queerness through the appearance of bodies, as this process makes invisible the queerness of femmes and other mislabeled bodies (Xhonneux, "Performing Butler" 299). Mia Mingus further challenges this linking of "femme" to ableist performances of fashion and beauty in order to center her queer of color body's lived experience of disability, reclaiming bodies that are coded as ugly, and that are therefore "*magnificent*." Because in *Gifts* these perceptual codes for queerness are unavailable, we rely on our narrator to disclose information regarding her own appearance (and desires), which time and again she withholds.

This withholding, however, need not presuppose a default assumption of straightness but might rather stand in for the unstated existence of a textual world that is already coded as queer. Rather than understanding the narrator as straight until labeled as otherwise, the narrative strategy of refusing this information creates an alternative to this normative reading practice, altogether avoiding the overwrought narrative act of coming out. Jack Halberstam identifies this refusal to name queerness within Harry Dodge and Silas Howard's 2001 independent film, *By Hook or by Crook*. Halberstam observes how the film's characters occupy a series of public spaces—cafes, clubs, stores, residences, hotels—wherein they are never forced to justify or explain their complex genders or label their sexual orientations, a narrative strategy that "effectively *universalizes queerness* within this specific cinematic space" (94). Halberstam further clarifies that the universality achieved by the film is not the same tactic of mainstream productions, which represent queer subcultures as being "just like everyone else," watering down queer experience in order to produce films that match every other Hollywood feature's aesthetic appeal to mass audiences (94). *By Hook or by Crook*, Halberstam reveals, "actually manages to tell a queer story that is more than a queer story by refusing to acknowledge the existence of a straight world . . . represent[ing] a truly localized place of opposition—an opposition, moreover, that is to be found in committed performances of perversity, madness, and friendship" (94). *Gifts*, accordingly, offers a literary model of HIV caregiving that builds sexual and gender nonconforming models of kinship without having to overtly label itself as queer. Like the other texts I analyze throughout this book, Brown's offers an ongoing model of how disability can bring queer and trans bodies together through the exchange of mutual care, in ways that are influenced by the—even unnamed—presence of sexual and gender nonconforming exchange. Paradoxically, in omitting overt labels of sexual and gender identity, queerness emerges in layered ways to encompass broad and unfixed models of intimacy between friends. Xhonneux, for instance, considers the absence of gender markers in Brown's fiction as a strategy that creates identity as a work in progress for the reader rather than fixing gender into a stable, binary, or normative set of assumptions ("Performing Butler" 305). Xhonneux notes, "Next to their looks, motivations, and names, the gender of Brown's protagonists is another means of characterization that is rarely mentioned explicitly. Xhonneux identifies this withholding of information as a "strategy" which "has the potential to liberate the reader from predetermined beliefs concerning gender and sexuality" (*Rebecca* 17). Brown's caregiving narrative can be read as one such cultural text that places queer subjectivity at its universal center, making space for unfixed sexualities, genders, and intimate caregiving relationships. These relationships and their representations in literature respond to HIV by expanding models for family, intimacy, and other queer kinships. Brown's depictions of HIV caregiving thus also widen literary possibilities for narrating sexuality and gender, and for narrating the openness of the connective relationships disability kinships may create. These narrative tactics not only are useful in depicting early HIV caregiving activism but continue to model fluid possibilities for queer and trans expression.

Brown's seemingly unintentional but arguably deliberate linguistic maneuvering, moreover, is not restricted to *Gifts*. Much of Brown's fiction rejects outright naming in favor of more intricate pronoun use and gendering practices that may go unnoticed by readers of her deceptively minimalist writing. For instance, in *Annie Oakley's Girl* (1993), the second-person pronoun, "you," often replaces gendered pronouns that would fix identity onto a given subject. In depicting queer sex in her short story "Folie A Deux" from this collection, Brown evades the use of gendered language through the use of this "you": "you had told me how you liked the leanness of my body, the way the ribs were hard and near the surface of my skin, and the spaces between them soft and giving" (52). Brown's "you" resists reinforcing essentialist tropes of femininity as requiring certain kinds of genitals or cliché descriptors. Queerness, by extension, is tied not only to the sex acts exchanged between two bodies but to experiences like caregiving that allow for a fluid expression of intimacies, genders, and desires. In an interview with Matthew Stadler, Brown explains her use of this "you": "In a lot of the stuff I wrote in the late '70s and early '80s—the I-You narratives in *Evolution of Darkness* and the sections of *The Terrible Girls* written then—there was a very specific person I was addressing in my mind, a girlfriend with whom I was obsessed" (8). In the interview, Brown traces the progression of this literary strategy from initially addressing girlfriends to moving toward broader considerations beyond her personal experiences of love and loss: "Now I am interested in the notion that there's some huge, amorphous 'You'—God or longing or the past—that I'm addressing. Which was probably also what I was seeking from those poor, decent-but-only-human girlfriends I got so insane about back then" (8). Reading this fluid "you" in connection to *Gifts* resists the fixing of identity implied by the very act of naming and, correlatively, of essentializing language or gender within her work; the narrative gaps where Brown omits naming/queerness expands preconceptions of who might be included within this second-person pronoun's address.

Brown's use of the second-person pronoun further creates an openness to her writing that supports a reading of *Gifts*' narrator's desires in fluid, queer ways. This "you" connects the unnamed narrator to Brown-the-author, another process of naming invited by the openness of this text. Sarah Brophy's reading of *Gifts* complicates the literary reach of this "you" by positioning it as an indication of Brown's authorial proximity to the personas she creates. Brophy depicts *Gifts* as "a fictionalized memoir" (115), "written from the perspective of a lesbian caring for people with AIDS" (115). While no concrete textual evidence supports Brophy's observation that the narrator is "a lesbian," she draws this conclusion by regarding the narrator as a "fictionalized (but autobiographically based)" (116) version of Brown. Though it does not call any overt attention to itself as such, the narrator's lesbianism serves as the starting point of Brophy's analysis, which puts into practice Halberstam's model of the universal queer. By reading queerness as foundational both to Brown as an author and to Brown's text as a queer cultural object, Brophy upsets straight reading practices that assume heterosexuality as a literary default. Ann Cvetkovich's reading of *Gifts* also supports that

Brown "queers" caretaking by nontraditionally practicing its gendered roles in "in butch ways" (226). Cvetkovich reads Brown's narrator as both queer and as butch, which further challenges the practice of assuming default heterosexuality or gender normativity for characters who do not explicitly proclaim these attributes. Cvetkovich connects the narrator's queer gender to the literary impact of her emotional withholding: "there is no easy sentimentality about *The Gifts of the Body* or the caretaker it depicts; yet it is also a deeply affecting novel, producing feeling in a style reminiscent of *Stone Butch Blues*'s emotional untouchability, where the feelings are hard won because they are so often fended off in service to others" (226). Withholding the naming of the narrator and her queerness actually enhances rather than undercuts the caregiving intimacies that structure the text: the narrator's withholding practices could also be read as setting the boundaries that allow for her emotional labor to be given in open, connective ways that support reciprocity in caregiving rather than risk burnout (Cvetkovich 226). Through an understated butch narrative expression of queer feeling as an asset to providing support, *Gifts* not only breaks from the desexualized norms of the caregiving narrative but also locates caregiving as part of this historical archive of HIV activism (Cvetkovich 237). Caregiving is rendered through literature as a form of queer activism, as a service that need not be undervalued as less transformative than direct action or street protest. Brown's narrative urges the reader to identify the gendered labor and activist potential of caregiving, valuing domestic kinds of frontline work that are less frequently acknowledged as such.

As a work of literature, this text offers an ongoing model of disability kinship that bonds sick and nonconforming bodies together through caregiving activism. The narrative of *Gifts* restores value to caregiving as a potentially reciprocal act that creates chosen family in response to HIV. Intimate, mutual connections are built through caregiving relationships and are then represented through narrative. Returning to Brown's literary depictions of care offers a disability narrative of caregiving-as-activism that continues in recognizing the transformative practice of caregiving within contemporary queer and trans disability movements. Although the narrator's queer gender and sexuality are not discussed overtly, her desires are nevertheless expressed through her connections to her clients, albeit in subtle ways. Like the friendship of "A Good Man," these bonds are not consummated or defined through fixed or essentialist definitions of sex. Brophy, for instance, regards the relationship between the narrator and her gay client, Rick, as a queer exchange. With Rick, queerness is expressed not merely through the provision of care and affection but through the exchange of fluids. This swapping of bodily fluids in the exchange of care includes types of intimate contact beyond sex alone (Delany, *Times Square* 90; Rifkin 36). In bringing bodies close enough to absorb each other's fluids, Brown constructs a bond between the narrator and her care recipients that also creates a textual intimacy between the narrator and her reader. Xhonneux suggests that this strategy of bodily intimacy might also serve to challenge readers' own serophobia and ableist assumptions upon reading depictions of contact (*Rebecca* 181). By trading sweat, Rick and the narrator can express their passion for one another through labor, again rendering caregiving a mutual and passionate process that blurs gender and sexual lines (Brophy, *Witnessing* 116). Eroticizing physical acts beyond "genital sexuality" (Cvetkovich 223), intimate queer bonds are established through gestures of care. Brown represents HIV kinships to expand gendered and essentialist understandings of what might constitute *sex*, and by extension, her narrative broadens the relations between bodies to expand what might constitute care (Cvetkovich 226). Queer caregiving, like queer sex, allows participants to redefine their gender and sexual positions by unhinging caregiving from predetermined norms. Rather than defining sex narrowly as requiring orgasm, certain body parts, or the presence of fluids, the type of contact that builds queer kinships through care yields a broad range of fluids that can be central to or can transcend representations of "intercourse." Just as the text presents the narrator's queerness and her gender in an open, unfixed way, the narrative representation of HIV caregiving offers models of nonconventionally sexual or other kinds of nonsexual but highly intimate relationship building. Brown's early HIV caregiving depictions provide ongoing narrative possibilities for representing the fluid intimacies formed in response to disability. These textual intimacies challenge the apparent simplicity of the narrator's writing style and the (lack of) personal information she discloses.

These queer disability kinships shared between the narrator and Rick can further be read toward better understanding the other caregiving relationships in this narrative. Brophy regards this relationship between Rick and the narrator as the beacon of queerness within Brown's text; Brophy therefore laments the return to heteronormative kinship models at the narrative's conclusion. Brophy posits how, in returning Connie's body and the locus of mourning from the narrator to Connie's biological children, Brown's ending "risks re-installing the nuclear family at the centre" (116). Yet, Brophy's reading dismisses the queerness inherent to Connie's biological family, as her other primary caregivers are her gay son and his partner, complicating the relationship between the queer (female) outsider and the queer (male) kin that together compose Connie's caregiving team. Brophy's reading of *Gifts* nevertheless creates an opportunity for interpreting *Gifts* as a queer text against the heteronormative caregiving and familial structures within which it operates. *Gifts* models how rather than relying upon single overworked primary caregivers, people living with HIV constructed caregiving teams from a variety of friends, family, lovers, volunteers, and professionals (DeLombard 351). This queer formation of a caregiving team that combines chosen and biological family is centered in Sarah Liss's 2013 publication, *Army of Lovers: A Community History of Will Munro*. Munro died of brain cancer in 2010, and his care team consisted of family and friends who, as Liss points out, belong to a generation that did not lose many kin to AIDS (107). This generational experience of caring for Munro can thus be connected back to Brown's narrative models of early HIV caregiving that blend biological family with queer and trans community care. Returning to Brown's work represents queer and trans kinship formations as a critical form of disability activism that extends early HIV caregiving across space and time.

The Gift of Names

In this section, I look specifically to practices of naming to connect early HIV narratives to ongoing disability kinships in the present. I read Brown's narrative as part of a larger ongoing literary and cultural project of naming disability kinships from the early years of HIV toward bringing them into contemporary disability movements. This ongoing process of naming HIV in relationship to disability can become a narrative act of collective remembering (Bride 2017; Bryan-Wilson, *Fray* 197, 250; "Art and Activism" 2008). The NAMES quilt, for example, centers this memorial process of naming that connects caregiving to mourning (Xhonneux, *Rebecca* 187; Bryan-Wilson, *Fray* 195). Queer critiques of this quilt also acknowledge the limits of the project in politicizing death, while nevertheless pointing to the importance the names of the dead hold can hold for the living (McRuer, "Disability" 59). In his discussion of the memorial practice of naming within the Black Lives Matter movement, C. Riley Snorton identifies the act of naming as "securing the existence of black and trans people in the present and into the future. The practice of remembering and saying their names is also a demand for new structures for naming that evince and eviscerate the conditions that continually produce black and trans death" (195). The representation of naming in *Gifts* renders memory and memorialization as another important form of care. The collective significance of these naming practices in *Gifts* is manifested through Roy, a resident of one of the dismal apartment buildings that house many of the narrator's clients. Upon being introduced to Roy, we learn from the narrator that he has come of age in a series of underfunded institutional settings including this one. When they meet in the elevator, Roy performs an uncanny feat of reciting the first and last names of all the building's past and present residents for the narrator. Although we never become privy to the narrator's own name, an eerie moment transpires when she discloses it to Roy: "I told him my name and he made this spitting sound; it was him giggling. 'I know,' he said, like I'd just fallen for this incredibly funny joke. Then he said very seriously, 'I know you. I've seen you before'" (88). This chilling, almost gothic sensation is characteristic of much of Brown's larger corpus, which features haunting scenarios like finding oneself participating in a never-ending honeymoon or having one's studio apartment invaded by an infinitely multiplying pack of dogs. Conjuring sentiments of this horror genre of Brown's earlier work, the narrator relays the discomfort she derives from Roy's act of naming: "It felt weird to think of this guy watching me from the elevator when I'd been in the building before" (88). While throughout the text, our narrator is the one who occupies this omniscient position of sharing confidential details of her clients' private lives, she becomes protective and even feels violated in response to this act of naming.

In witnessing the narrator's emotional revulsion in response to being named by Roy, the reader, interestingly, can glean not the inappropriateness but rather the importance of Roy's naming practices. By experiencing discomfort in this act of exposure, the narrator undercuts her own position in disclosing the vulnerabilities of her clients, and correspondingly Brown also unsettles the casual voyeurism of the reader. Not only does the narrator experience unease from Roy's ability to remember an unusual number of names, but in relaying his mode of recitation, the narrator figures him as a grim reaper, summoning the residents toward their inescapable deaths. Brown presents naming as an act through which readers might begin to register some of the narrator's own discomforts with poverty and with disability. This moment also symbolizes the disjuncture between the narrator's understanding of HIV and her understanding of disability more broadly. She seems not to recognize HIV *as* disability, as her sensitivity in HIV caregiving does not translate to her respectful treatment of Roy. The reader is thus positioned to consider why the narrator feels sympathy for disabilities that result from illness rather than from intellectual or physical difference. As the narrator comes into contact with Roy via his presence within subsidized housing, Brown raises larger questions regarding how institutional care—in contrast to the community and familial care provided to clients like the middle-class Connie—is itself disabling.

Roy's character thus begins to undermine some of the secrecy and seamless authority held by our narrator, as well as her proximity to our author. Feeling increasingly uncomfortable with Roy's performance, the narrator tries to disarm him through condescension: "'That's a lot of names,' I said. 'I know your name too,' he said. I felt my skin crawl" (90). As the narrator manages to relay this entire sequence without actually disclosing her own name, the narrator's observations of Roy reinforce the narrative's mounting connections between naming, intimacy, and memory (D. Levine 3–4; 35). Andrew, another HIV caregiver who is also present (and named) during this interaction in the elevator, counters the narrator's fears of Roy by regarding his disability and his person as having value in spite of his relegation to this apartment complex. Andrew characterizes Roy as an "archivist" (91), joking not only that Roy documents the building's tenancy but that "he also does the obits" (91). When the narrator condescendingly observes how "it's amazing he remembers all the names" (91), Andrew sighs, lamenting, "It's nice someone does" (91). In relaying this failure of memory, Brown's disability narrative becomes part of this archive, document-ing the magnitude of a loss so vast that it cannot be named.

This process of naming also (de)codes the narrator's queerness and how it informs her caregiving connections to her clients. Naming, again, is not an inci-dental occurrence in the text but an act of disclosure that signals the intimate relationships that form caregiving kinships. Naming becomes the process that connects early HIV archives of body self-determination to queer and trans dis-ability activism in the present. Following her meeting with Roy, the narrator is introduced to a new client named Frances Martin. This same haunting apart-ment building provides the backdrop to another moment that, like the narra-tor's subtle exchange of understanding with Connie, could be read as queer. After introducing herself to her new client, he responds, "'I don't remember your name, but I know you.' He tried to raise his hand. I took it to shake. 'I'm Marty,' he said. But his name was supposed to be Francis, Francis Martin" (93). The dis-crepancy between the client's official name and the name he chooses poses a problem for the narrator, a dilemma linked to recognition: "'We've met before,' he insisted. 'Uh-huh,' I said vaguely. There was no point in trying to correct someone with dementia. He kept looking at me very intently. 'I was Carlos's friend,' he said. I was still shaking his hand, not getting it" (93). When the nar-rator overcomes her preconceptions about dementia to concede her own mem-ory's limitations, we learn that she has in fact met this man before. In yet another uncanny moment of recognition, she relates, "He clutched my hand to stop shak-ing. Then I remembered and I got a horrible chill. My skin prickled. 'Oh—right!' I said. 'Marty!'" (93). Through this skin-pricking sensation, the narrator recalls that this Marty is the same Marty who once struck the narrator as appear-ing "pear-shaped" and as having "baby fat on his face" (94). The narrator real-izes that the signs of Marty's illness are apparent only in having known Marty before he became sick: "If you saw him for the first time you might not think he was sick, just trim" (94). Naming exposes our narrator's relationship to body size and "trim-ness," while also making apparent her discomfort with Marty's ill-ness: "I tried to smile like it was nice to run into him again but it was horrify-ing" (94). Comparing this moment to her earlier discomfort at hearing her own name pronounced by Roy, the narrator again identifies her unease with disabil-ity through this process of naming and recognition: "I thought of how strange I felt when Roy told me he knew my name. It was nothing compared to what Marty must have felt" (96). Yet like Andrew, Marty does not share the narrator's assump-tion that the presence of disability should necessarily elicit a reaction of "horror." Instead, Marty calmly registers the narrator's reaction and attempts to alleviate her discomfort through further disclosure: "I saw him recognize the look on my face. But he was polite. He tried to make conversation" (94). Echoing the professional tone of the initial meeting between the narrator and Connie, small talk and "polite" conversation again stand in as textual buffers to the discomfort of witnessing suffering.

These passages, however, demonstrate the utility of reading Brown's work for what is *unsaid*, revealing textual possibilities for queer intimacy via HIV caregiving. These understated moments in the narrative are easy to miss but nonetheless significant in how they model ongoing disability kinships. As with the narrator's earlier interactions with Connie, this practice of "polite" conversation can bring about an unspoken acknowledgment of queerness. Once they commence their conversation, Marty and the narrator share a deceptively simple exchange that permits the mutual recognition of support. As the two discuss the caregiving relationship that existed between Marty and Carlos, a moment of identification transpires between them: "He looked at me again like he was checking me out. 'Have you ever had a friend like that?' 'Yes,' I said immediately" (98). Although on the surface the two appear to be politely discussing the nature of friendship, Marty's "checking [the narrator] out" and the narrator's "immediate" response recall the dyke-fag intimacies of "A Good Man." It is this rapid moment of queer identification, furthermore, that allows the narrator to provide genuine care to this client: "'It's nice to see you again too, Marty,' I said, and I meant it then. I felt something when I thought about Marty and Carlos" (94). Queerness, though unspoken, plays an integral role in buffering and naturalizing what could otherwise become a forced or awkward relationship between caregiver and recipient. Moving past the initial "politeness" apparent in this interaction, queer recognition becomes an elemental, if less readily discernable, component of Brown's text.

These brief queer exchanges are also significant in understanding the literary function of the emotional distance the narrator creates in depicting her clients, as well as the role of storytelling itself in separating her from those to whom she gives care. What Jennifer Blair terms Brown's "rhetoric of restraint" (523)—or absence of personal disclosure—creates a narrative gap within which to grapple with the cultural meanings of HIV and with readers' preconceptions about disability (Blair 533). The sparsity of personal disclosure points to the boundaries the narrator needs to maintain between herself and her clients, and it is thus interesting to read what happens when this capacity for boundedness and narrative remove is broken. For much of the plot, we can only speculate about the narrator's sexuality and personal life. We actually receive no information about her own partners until she encounters a new client named Keith. Unlike in previous chapters of *Gifts*, where clients are introduced in a humanizing and respectful manner, "The Gift of Sight" opens with a startling dose of judgment and distance: "This guy was the scariest to look at. This guy really looked like the plague" (117). Reflecting medical and media narratives of the 1980s that stigmatize disability as a gay plague by reducing people living with HIV to symptoms of contagion, the narrator suddenly becomes unable to perceive Keith outside of his symptoms. While the narrator remains most removed from this client, it is their detached relationship that ultimately allows the narrator to finally open up to her readers. Though the narrator is "frightened" (117) by the sores that cover Keith's body, it is while applying salve to Keith's wounds that the narrator at last begins to speak of her own personal life: "Part of it felt good, like a normal conversation you'd have with someone you met at a party or with a new neighbor. But also it was like there were four different people there. The two people having the normal conversation and the person touching the body with the salve and the person with the body with the sores" (121). This fractured intimacy forces the narrator away from the comfortably stoic role she assumes as a storyteller/caregiver. The personal distance that forms between her and Keith actually fosters some of the self-reflection conspicuously absent from the rest of the text. Our narrator's dissociative relationship to Keith's body thereby elimi-nates some of our own emotional distance from her. In touching this client's body, the narrator begins to concede her own limitations and guilt, revealing, "I hated myself for thinking that but I also kept telling myself that even if I wasn't feeling or thinking the right things, at least he was getting fed, at least he was getting his sheets changed, at least his kitchen was getting cleaned, at least his body was getting salve" (122). It is not until the narrator confronts the power imbalance inherent to caregiving that she becomes able to open up about her own inner life. In admitting that in spite of her best intentions, she still harbors insecurities and prejudices toward her clients, the narrator can finally disclose some her own experiences as well: "I started in on the salve. While I did it I told him about what I'd been up to that week, about a movie I'd gone to and hiking with Chris and a new string game I taught my cat" (123).

Though these details remain rather sparse, they provide a great wealth of information in comparison to the meager tidbits we receive up to this point, making us cherish even the smallest allusions to the narrator's personal life. As Valerie Miner observes in her review of *Gifts*, Brown's reader is intended to feel dissatisfied with the details we are given, producing a strong yearning to learn more about our narrator. Miner observers how "gradually the narrator emerges from the interstices as a self-contained, understated woman. We learn that she has a friend named Chris, has been to college, is planning to visit San Francisco and has lost someone close to AIDS. For the most part, this indirect self-presentation works, but occasionally I wanted to know more about her" (14). Miner, perhaps not so well versed in the details of Brown's own life, takes her depiction of "Chris" as the narrator's "friend." However, any reader familiar with Brown's biography would glean that the Chris in the text alludes to the Chris in *Gifts*' acknowledgments, which read, "To Chris Galloway: Thanks for the gift of the heart" (165). This acknowledgment of Galloway's care leads us to wonder why this gift is so heavily veiled in the rest of the text, failing to constitute a more

overt recognition of a relationship between the narrator and her long-term lesbian lover, who likely provides daily support upon coming home from her job.
Reading the caregiving role of Chris, even though she is only mentioned in passing, widens the queer intimacies in this novel into those spaces unseen in the
plot, like the domestic. As Brown reveals in an interview with Carol Guess, the
care she receives from Galloway allows her to confront sadness through her literary work, another kind of labor that creates the book itself through the writing process of authoring a memoir (or novelization of personal experience?) yet
is invisible in the world of the text. Brown reflects, "I am also very very fortunate that my partner of 15 years is a great person, both very independent and
very loving. That I have been able to make a home with her has, I think, enabled
me to keep living and writing, especially writing really sad stuff that, were I not
in this good relationship, might just sink me down to somewhere I couldn't come
back from" (6). The near absence of such a character from *Gifts* raises interesting auto/biographical questions about why a character of such importance in
Brown's own life did not translate into its narrative adaptation. This gap also
questions why the public kinships formed through this care work are not brought
into narrative conversation with those that sustain that work through home.
Unlike the HIV romance of "A Good Man" that develops out of a preexisting
care relationship, explicitly queer bonds between intimate lovers and friends in
Gifts are demonstrated only by secondary (male) characters such as Marty and
Carlos or Tony and Joe. In keeping a professional distance from her clients (and
from her readers), the narrator omits herself from the queer kinships central to
her own story.

It is thus curious why this gap in the narrative occurs and what can be gleaned
from reading this literary omission in the present. The distance that Brown estab-
lishes through this withholding might speak to the gap felt by younger contemporary readers who were not personally affected by exchanging care and
losing kin during this historical period that *Gifts* memorializes. Because the book
was initially published for a wide audience who might not have personally taken
part in HIV caregiving activism, its transmission to a generation of queer and
trans readers who would have likely formed HIV caregiving kinships had they
been older/alive in the 1980s and early 1990s could also reinterpret this gap
between narrator and reader as opportunity to bring these models into ongoing
disability organizing. Brown's narrative shift from short story to novel could also
reflect the difference between providing care through nonprofit or other hierar-
chically structured caregiving networks and providing it through those that are
collectively organized or part of one's own preexisting networks. These differences
might also reflect the exchange of money for caregiving labor in *Gifts* in contrast
to the kinds of romantic, anticapitalist exchanges of "A Good Man." The narrator's
supervisor Margaret provides a noteworthy exception to these representations of
providing care from a professional and emotional distance. Margaret's name

appears multiple times throughout the text, though we do not actually meet her until the end of the narrative, when we discover that she too has become ill with AIDS. It is not until Margaret's disclosure that the narrator understands for the first time how it feels to know someone who is diagnosed with AIDS rather than meeting someone because they are already sick: "there is always a hole when someone died" (157), the narrator realizes while thinking of Margaret; "it was always in the middle of people" (157). Though nearly burnt out on a professional level, suddenly the narrator also comes to understand HIV care more personally. Margaret's disclosure prompts the narrator to seek comfort in Connie, complicating their unidirectional relationship as caregiver and care recipient: "I held her longer than usual. I kept holding her and couldn't let go. When she felt me holding her like that she started to stroke my hair. Her hands were thin but stronger than I thought" (135). Connie's unexpected strength and support allow the narrator to acknowledge how the detachment that exists between herself and her clients (and by extension, her readers) becomes a protective shield that falsely separates herself from others—and falsely separates the disabled body from the able-bodied—under the guise of professionalism. At the novel's conclusion, the narrator (and therefore the reader) ultimately recognizes how reciprocal relationships are established through the vulnerable labor not only of providing care but also of receiving it.

Sweet Personal Friendships

In this final section, I analyze how Brown's own queerness codes her depictions of HIV as something generative of connection and mutual desire across gender and sexual lines. Toward this book's larger project of reimagining disability by bringing early HIV narratives into the present, I consider how in spite of—and arguably even because of—the omission of overt queer representation, *Gifts* ultimately renders HIV caregiving as a process that can create expansive, fluid kinships in support of mutual vulnerability and interdependence. Brown's tactic both of coding and of structuring around the narrator's queerness allows contemporary readers to use this textual gap toward the intergenerational witnessing of ongoing disability activisms for body self-determination from early HIV caregiving into the present. Contemporary readers can also interpret these understated exchanges of queer solidarity between these now-historical characters as signifying the power of coming together to care for one another to cope with death and stigma. The narrative distance with which Brown represents this exchange of care initially veils but eventually affirms the significance of queer relational models in providing reciprocity in caregiving. Queer kinship models are not often named but nevertheless structure much of the interconnectedness between the narrator and her clients throughout the text. Though *Gifts* cryptically codes its narrator's sexuality and gender presentation, interviews with

Brown demonstrate her unyielding commitment to writing from within queer literary community. Brown explains, "I feel connected to a community in Seattle. Which for me means sweet personal friendships and excitement about each other's work" (7). Brown's stated commitment to queerness in her writing is not merely about the content of the work but about its community-driven production: "I also feel, politically rather than aesthetically, the importance of being a writer who is an out lesbian, connecting myself to that community. I hate closeted writers" (7). Brown discusses how queerness often exists oppositionally to mainstream publishing, manifesting instead as "D.I.Y culture. Small presses. 'Zines. Work that does not attempt to synthesize or bring things together, but insists on its own incompleteness, its own—if I can yank a word back into another, older meaning—'queerness'" (8). Brown identifies independently published, do-it-yourself formulations as ideal outlets for expressing queer ways of relating. As Brown reveals, "I hate how dismissive mainstream arts, money, and power are of work by and about out lesbians. I am excited about small presses and experimental writing and feel I and my work fit in there more happily than elsewhere" (7). While "A Good Man" is published by City Lights, an independent small press that prides itself as "a champion of progressive thinking, fighting against the forces of conservatism and censorship," *The Gifts of the Body* is published by HarperCollins, a mainstream venue whose wider readership may have cost the book's potential lesbian content (Schulman, "Guess" 16). Thus, the contrast between the queerly published "A Good Man" and the more mainstream *Gifts* may actually mirror the greater normalizing trends of cultural industries at large. These trends include the marginalization of depictions of disability that convey the mutuality of care in queer and nonnormative ways. In a British review of Brown's autobiographical *Excerpts from a Family Medical Dictionary* (2003), Ali Smith also discusses *Gifts*, arguing that Brown displays "a sense of truthfulness not found in the work of many writers" (1). Smith points out that reviews of Brown's work are characterized by epithets like "unflinching" (1), which consistently fail to "do justice" (1) to her literary accomplishments. As Smith asserts, "Brown is a great writer, a quiet, uneasy trailblazer, who hasn't really received her due of critical attention either here or in the States. Her latest book will probably also be labeled unflinching" (1). *Gifts* also exists within a larger body of women's HIV caregiving including Amy Hoffman's *Hospital Time*, wherein Hoffman, "without flinching" (Vaid ix), describes her relationship to her dying best friend Michael. Published through Duke University Press in 1997, this autobiography's release by way of academic publishing suggests the filling of a gap in literary markets. However, rather than merely lament mainstream publishing as removing lesbian content or antinormative meanings from Brown's work, these textual gaps actually create literary space to reframe disability as creating fluid kinships for sexual and gender self-determination into the present: Brown's literature invites an emerging generation of queer and trans readers to occupy the narrative space held by this textual openness and by the fluidity of early HIV caregiving and the queer exchanges it invites us to decode.

Through this narrative process of naming and withholding, *The Gifts of the Body* reframes caregiving as a fluid and potentially reciprocal act that can link present-day readers to early HIV activism and its memorialization. Unlike in "A Good Man," caregiving in *Gifts* is provided as a professional service rather than as an extension of queer love between friends. Nevertheless, the intimacies formed through the narrator's paid labor demonstrate the potential of caregiving's "gifts" in expanding queer relational models through the intimate and mutual exchange of care. Chapter 5, the final chapter in this book, considers the representation of biological family caregiving in Jamaica Kincaid's *My Brother* to raise further questions about narrative withholding in connection to sexuality, forced migration, and family trauma. In tracing these caregiving networks across transnational borders and prison spaces, this book's final chapter will consider the capacity of caregiving narratives to reframe definitions of home and family toward decriminalization and prison abolition. Like Brown's narrative withholding, Kincaid's depictions of caring and not caring for her brother again raise questions about why an autobiographer would conceal rather than share narrative information in her memoir. Moving from this investigation of Brown's emotional withholding as caregiving labor, the final chapter will again question the reliability of our autobiographer toward analyzing the queer interconnectivities and mutual vulnerabilities made apparent in narrating early HIV caregiving into the present.

CHAPTER 5

Queering Customs

UNBURYING CARE IN *MY BROTHER* AND ACE

Like Rebecca Brown's deceptively straightforward narration, Jamaica Kincaid's early HIV caregiving autobiography conceals more personal information than it provides. This chapter revisits Kincaid's narrative tactics for depicting the reciprocity of care when trust is broken by the first-person autobiographer. As with those of *The Gifts of the Body* in chapter 4, Kincaid's textual omissions offer a narrative model of disability kinship that links early HIV caregiving to contemporary queer and trans body self-determination. Close-reading this text reveals how HIV caregiving can bring bodies together across spatial and sexual lines, building intimacies and documenting them as memoir, albeit unreliably. Building from my earlier chapters' analyses of how chosen family forms in response to disability, this final chapter reads caregiving literature to uncover how Kincaid's withholding narrative style connects representations of HIV kinship to ongoing strategies for decriminalization. This chapter revisits Kincaid's 1997 memoir *My Brother* alongside the work of the Bedford Prison activist collective AIDS Counseling and Education (ACE). These archives complicate narrative divisions between gay and straight, here and elsewhere, inside prison and out. While Kincaid's diasporic narrative undercuts the policing of national borders, ACE's caregiving activism breaks down storytelling processes that imagine prison spaces as existing apart from the communities from which prisoners are taken. Early HIV caregiving narratives thus provide ongoing antiracist, anticolonial, abolitionist strategies for replacing prisons with more caring forms of anticarceral justice.

SECRET WEAPONS

I open this chapter with an investigation of current movements toward HIV decriminalization and prison abolition. In the sections that follow, I then close-read Kincaid's *My Brother* to link the present to early HIV caregiving narratives and their strategies for resisting state and medical violence. Finally, I return to archives of early HIV prison organizing, bringing together film, literature, oral history, and documentary genres to trace caregiving kinships in response to disability. Revisiting these early models of HIV caregiving offers ongoing narrative strategies for HIV decriminalization. Because the outcome of HIV stigma in the present continues to lead to incarceration, storytelling remains a tool for ending the violence of prisons and the police. This narrative process exposes connections between disability, racism, and incarceration, as critical theorists have established the ongoing effects of colonialism on individual bodies. In their preface to *Disability Incarcerated* (2014), Liat Ben-Moshe, Chris Chapman, and Allison C. Carey discuss the links between seemingly unrelated forms of institutionalization as nursing homes, long-term care facilities, prisons, and detention centers. They unite these various forms of confinement by tracing a process by which emerging institutions continue the function of the older systems they replace. They discuss, for instance, the Sixties Scoop, wherein indigenous children were removed from their communities during the period following the official closure of residential schools (Ben-Moshe et al. x; Sinclair 66). The authors connect this ongoing national project of cultural genocide and forced assimilation to narratives of disability, arguing that "the ongoing institutionalization of these survivors' children [is] sometimes now politically rationalized through the dividing practices of disability rather than race" (Ben-Moshe et al. x; Sinclair 78). HIV narratives, in particular, evidence how storytelling about disability continues to be leveraged by the state to justify ongoing colonial practices. As Syrus Ware, Joan Ruzsa, and Giselle Dias argue, "the brutality of the attempted genocide of Indigenous people has had, and continues to have, a disabling affect. This experience of disability is exacerbated by the PIC [Prison Industrial Complex]" (166). HIV archives, however, also document the long history of black and indigenous resistance to this policing of nonconforming bodies into the present (Kelly and Orsini; Sinclair 67). While cultural narratives can be used to stigmatize HIV, HIV narratives can conversely offer interventions into processes of state violence by supporting bodily sovereignty. Kincaid's memoir can be read as an early HIV narrative that provides an ongoing model for continuing to challenge the institutional regulation of queer and gender nonconforming bodies through disability kinships and their narrative representations.

Bringing early HIV caregiving narratives into the present offers a model for generations who are still impacted by the early years of HIV activism but were then still too young (or not alive yet) in the 1980s and early 1990s to find HIV kinships. Looking back at these archives of desire and loss presents ongoing narrative strategies for queer and trans youth to continue to connect with these legacies of HIV activism and to engage with the disability kinship possibilities they offer. Moving early HIV caregiving archives across time and out of the past, Adam Garnet Jones, a queer filmmaker and writer of Cree and Métis ancestry, reanimates the early HIV archive to connect his own generational experience of HIV narratives as a teenager in the early 1990s to current conversations of resisting ongoing colonialization. Garnet Jones's 2008 short film *Secret Weapons* pays homage to experimental Canadian gay filmmaker Mike Hoolbloom's 1993 short film *Frank's Cock*. This source text, *Frank's Cock*, divides the screen into four quadrants, and each channel presents varied types of cinematic images. Hoolbloom's viewer simultaneously watches gay porn, scientific footage of cells, and a talking head monologue about Frank, whose relationship with the narrator is relayed against a backdrop of recollections about such familiarities as Canadian national radio and marathon sex. Hoolbloom ends this monologue by quoting Frank's hospital musing that "the body does not believe in progress. Its religion is the present not the future." "He's always saying crazy things like that," interjects the talking head from the top right quadrant of the frame, "so nothing's really changed. Except. He's dying. And I'm going to miss him. He was the best friend I ever had." In referencing Hoolbloom's source film while "reinterpreting the framework of the four channels as a digital medicine wheel," Garnet Jones occupies the fourth quadrant of his own frame to conjure HIV history in order to relay his "experiences of growing up under the fear of AIDS in the 1990s, and of the cultural loss and grief that has cycled through the Native community since colonization began." (See fig. 5.1.) *Secret Weapons* opens with Garnet Jones's narrative of mourning and loss that eulogizes "the missing generation. The heroes stolen by AIDS, the great minds murdered and paralyzed by residential schools, by the justice system." Garnet Jones brings these forms of state violence together into the present across narrative space and time (Kafer 36–37; Clare, *Brilliant* 87; Edelman, *No Future* 75; Berlant 58). Because the images and animations displayed in the other three quadrants that accompany the filmmaker are community-based collaborations between artists, activists, and youth, Garnet Jones presents the channels in tandem as "creating a moving portrait of a community, my own network of 'Secret Weapons.'" This portrait of collective support thus uses Hoolbloom's source text to link early HIV archives with youth movements, an address to second and third generations of survivors. By extending his influence's narrative format into a community portrait, Garnet Jones reframes disability as forming ongoing kinships in support of body self-determination.

Garnet Jones's film further connects these contemporary kinships to the early HIV friendships of Hoolbloom's text, and to the older generations of HIV activists to whose work Garnet Jones responds. *Secret Weapons* creates a lineage with early HIV archives to demonstrate the ongoing impact of disability narratives and their reframing in the present. Garnet Jones narrates his own experience of coming of age in a generation too young to have participated in early HIV activism but old enough to learn about HIV through stigmatizing mainstream media narratives linking queerness to inevitable decline. Garnet Jones uses Hoolbloom's

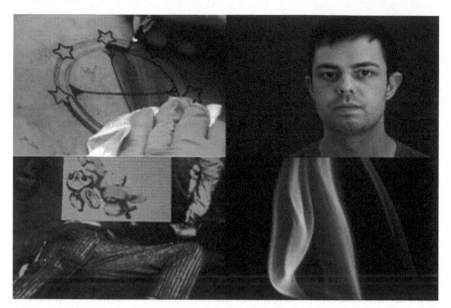

Figure 5.1. A still from *Secret Weapons* (2008) by Adam Garnet Jones. Courtesy of Adam Garnet Jones.

intimate style of confession to discuss HIV and colonization, creating resistance by confronting the two in tandem. "I woke up with a sore throat this morning," opens Garnet Jones's monologue, linking his own "shitty" feelings about HIV stigma to broader interlinked processes of colonization and loss: "I feel like I'm always in mourning," Garnet Jones continues, "and I wonder if that's intentional. Part of somebody's plan. I wonder if it's a tactic. A way to solve the fag problem, the Indian problem. I wonder if they want us . . . to grieve without stopping until that's all we are . . . grief that only comes from more grief and history." Connecting the history of AIDS losses to the history of Canada, Garnet Jones recalls being fourteen years old in the 1990s:

> This was it, if I was going to be a faggot, I would die of AIDS or worse. I didn't know what worse was but I spent a lot of time imagining it. But it didn't matter because in that moment, my fourteen-year-old body, my fourteen-year-old brain said yes to death. Said yes to a life of shame, of hiding in corners, of loveless affairs, of dying skinny and alone in a hospital, because that's what everything told me it would be like. And even faced with all that shit, with death, I knew that it would be worth it, to open up my body and my life up to danger just to be able to live and maybe fall in love.

In framing death as "worth it" and as the tradeoff for experiencing life, Garnet Jones then concedes that survival is possible only as an intergenerational, collective process. "If we're going to survive," Garnet Jones concludes, "we need to own each other, we need to know that if one of us goes down, there's going to be someone else to take our place, and someone else to take our place after that. And maybe then we'll stop being those people that the world wants us to be. Those vanishing people, those sick people, those weak people. I'm ready for that. What do you say?" *Secret Weapons* thus includes its viewer in forming communities of care in response to HIV in order to disrupt colonial genocide. This text models the narrative impact of bringing early HIV archives into contemporary reinterpretation for generations who did not directly experience these early losses but can draw on their records to form ongoing HIV families by connecting past and present.

This model of intergenerational HIV storytelling from Garnet Jones's film reframes HIV narratives as supporting body sovereignty through the formation of disability kinships. This narrative process transmits stories of nonconforming bodies surviving across generations. These stories document the creation of caregiving networks autonomously from, and in opposition to, the violence of the state. By returning to the early HIV caregiving of Kincaid's memoir, moving the past into the present again offers a model of representing disability kinships to counter the white settler project at a narrative level by challenging the function of national borders themselves. As a wide range of scholarship has shown, national borders extend colonial violence, creating further access barriers to care (Loyd et al.18; Mirza 218; Ben-Moshe, "Alternatives" 260). In sanctioning state violence against black indigenous and racialized bodies, borders further impede health-care access by narrating border crossings as a potential site of infection (Romero-Cesareo 106; D'Adesky 17). Border narratives are leveraged by the state to justify violence against already marginalized bodies through narratives of contagion (Baynton 33; Farrell 84–85; Showalter, *Sexual* 4; Wald 82; Cohen 139; Hartman 86). As Maria Ruiz argues, those vulnerable to detention or deportation through the act of accessing health care are the same populations for whom state violence creates an escalating risk of HIV infection (51; Farmer 183). However, rather than increase medical access for those without state support, border narratives frame HIV as justification for more stringent policing and incarceration as a way of preventing disability (J. Epstein, *Altered* 169–71; Wald 152). Countering such narratives of disability-as-threat and of illness as emerging always from elsewhere, HIV literature holds the potential to offset these narratives of criminalization through the representation of care from early HIV activism into the present.

Border narratives of HIV caregiving also offer an archive of queer and trans intimacies and models of disability kinship that expand conventional relationship structures. Kincaid's memoir can be read alongside queer theoretical work that connects HIV caregiving activism to queer and trans narratives of creating activist communities in support of health-care access and body self-determination. In *Compañeros: Latino Activists in the Face of AIDS*, Jesus

Ramirez-Valles presents a history of Latinx HIV support groups on the U.S.-Mexico border. Countering whitewashed and appropriative versions of HIV history (7, 118), Ramirez-Valles depicts these HIV groups as a critical venue for cruising and for solidifying friendships between trans women and cis gay men (111). These relationships formed though HIV caregiving, moreover, created not merely traditional couplings but a network of *compañeros*, providing alternatives to heteronormative relationship models that privilege the nuclear family above other types of kinships, friendships, and community networks (Ramirez-Valles 158). These deep bonds, argues Ramirez-Valles, became the organizational hub and energizing force essential to providing access to HIV education (158). Care, these kinship networks demonstrate, is a process not merely of giving but also of self-understanding (Ramirez-Valles 138–39). Community involvement, Ramirez-Valles identifies, is as much about learning about oneself as it is about helping others or creating social change. HIV education therefore centers the process of creating kinships to resist gender and racial oppression (Ramirez-Valles 138–39). This legacy of kinship formations and the expansion of family norms through border activism is also taken up within Karma Chávez's *Queer Migration Politics*. Chávez argues that critiques of the border can create coalitional gestures between documented and undocumented queers: anti-border activism form family and relations with others who are not partners or lovers (77). Such networks of seeing family more broadly critique the usefulness of marriage as a form of state recognition by imagining the undoing of borders (Chávez 145). Such an undoing, Chávez explains, indicates queer migration activists asking not just for what they think they can get but for what they want, countering capitalist scarcity as an act of care (48). Following Gloria Anzaldúa's tactic of envisioning the border as "a more heterogeneous transnational space of identity formation" (qtd. in Castillo and Cordoba 3; Chávez 11), HIV border narratives expand family through the decriminalization of migration. In the section that follows, I revisit Kincaid's caregiving memoir to present an ongoing model of HIV kinships that reframe disability through narratives of decolonization through the exchange of care.

A Monument to Boring Conventionality

In this section, I begin my reading of Kincaid's *My Brother*, an auto/biography that connects caregiving to experiences of family displacement and forced migration. As scholars of feminist autobiography argue, the genre is as much about the other as it is about the self; the narrator depicts her brother's life to talk about her own experience and vice versa, relaying auto/biographical subjects as relational and interdependent (Hallas 26; Watson 29–30; Miller 2; Freiwald 38). Close-reading this text alongside Jasbir Puar's theoretical work exposes the narrative process whereby BIPOC bodies transnationally are expected to live with debility and pain, rather than receive medical access or disability rights. As Puar argues, "what counts as a disability is already overdetermined by 'white fragility' on one side and the racialization of bodies that are expected to endure pain, suffering, and injury on the other" (*Right to Maim* xiv). Kincaid's narrative represents HIV kinships to reframe all bodies, even those living "without state recognition" (Puar, *Right to Maim* xvi), as deserving access to body self-determination (Puar, *Right to Maim* xxiv). This HIV caregiving memoir challenges these narratives that subject certain bodies to "expected" (Puar, *Right to Maim* xiv) debility. Though border anxiety is always "multidirectional" (Ruiz 39), narratives of contagion focus largely on crossings into but rarely out of U.S. borders. Kincaid counters this narrative practice through representations of caregiving. Kincaid begins her account of her brother Devon's experience of living with HIV by detailing her own migration away from the Caribbean. But rather than representing migration as a linear progression from one place to another, Kincaid shuttles between depictions of her brother's illness and recollections of her own childhood in Antigua. Because Kincaid remains removed from the persona she creates (Nikolas 59), I refer to her "narrator" as such to distinguish the narrator's perspective from that of Kincaid's authorial voice. Close-reading this text makes apparent how Kincaid's own voice emerges against rather than through her narrator's. In undercutting her own narrator's perspective, Kincaid renders failures in caregiving as connected to ongoing histories of colonialization.

It is through these unreliable gaps between author and persona that Kincaid's literary maneuvers unsettle cultural stories that normalize debility. While the narrator spends much time describing her brother's declining health, her narrative without much straightforward motivation lends equal weight to recounting the numerous insurrections between herself and her mother. The narrator explains that her mother's "love for her children when they are children is spectacular, unequalled I am sure in the history of a mother's love" (17). After presenting this grandiose claim, the narrator then portrays how her mother's "extraordinary ability of her love for her children . . . turn[s] into a weapon for their destruction" (53). We eventually come to learn that the narrator cannot forgive her mother for taking her out of school as a teenager to become a caregiver for her young siblings. The narrator explains that had "[her] life stayed on the path where [her] mother had set it" (74), the narrator would not have been able to pay from the United States for her brother's medications: "My brother would have been dead by now and . . . this act of my mother's [would have] been all that remained of my life" (74). The narrator also explains in impressive detail—and with much repetition—the care her mother provides while her brother is dying. These depictions are filled not so much with praise for her mother's ability to care for her dying son but rather with resentment for her mother's harm done to her daughter while her daughter lives. Caregiving, the narrator explains, is only provided by her mother when her children are dependent. This form of care impels the narrator to "remove [her]self" (20) from her mother's family and their needs, a feat the narrator can no longer accomplish once she learns her brother is dying. While the narrator wishes to keep her past at a geographical and emotional distance, her brother's disability prompts her to cross borders back into her family's reach.

As the plot unfolds, this gap between the author and narrator becomes more apparent. Kincaid continuously undercuts the narrator's resentments about her family and their need for care. Kincaid presents this story of Devon's disability to characterize her narrator's own dislocated understanding of kinship and home (48). The narrator remembers that, when she was growing up, "I decided that only people in Antigua died, that people living in other places did not die and as soon as I could, I would move somewhere else" (27). Although the trajectory of her brother's terminal diagnosis appears to support this juvenile belief, Kincaid's narrative actually fulfills the reverse function of illustrating how one cannot migrate away from disability (52). Mortality, which Kincaid attempts to escape upon leaving Antigua, effectively follows our heroine across borders, complicating her narrative of a seemingly impenetrable new life in Vermont.

Close-reading this family drama therefore opens ongoing narrative critiques of borders, of colonialism, and of "aftermaths of Atlantic chattel slavery" (Sharpe 2), as separating the members of Kincaid's family from the easy exchange of one another's care, even when Kincaid as a child was still living with them in Antigua. It is, in fact, Devon's disability that forces Kincaid to confront the border itself. Kincaid discusses her brother's lack of access to medication in Antigua, recalling a conversation with another HIV caregiver in Antigua who also maintains a diasporic identity as "a British woman of African descent" (48). In their readings of *My Brother*, Katherine Stanton identifies this other caregiver as an "AIDS activist" (49), and Sarah Brophy labels her a "fellow traveler" ("Angels in Antigua" 267): the narrator herself sparsely characterizes this woman as "a leader of workshops" (*My Brother* 48) whom she meets "at a workshop she was leading for people who wanted to volunteer to be AIDS counselors" (48). Kincaid's convoluted retelling of her interactions with this woman evidently maintains confusion about information identifying whether this woman is merely traveling to Antigua or whether she now lives there; whether this woman's workshops are activist, and what makes them so; and whether Kincaid herself becomes an activist by taking this training to provide HIV counseling as a form of care (or whether she begins providing HIV counseling, as this too is unmentioned either way). Remembering their conversation while "going through Customs" (48), Kincaid recounts how this woman recommends, "as if it were the most natural, obvious suggestion in the world, that I should take him to the United States for treatment" (48). In response to this apparently startling suggestion, Kincaid cites the border as the barrier to bringing her brother home: "I said, Oh, I am sure they wouldn't let him in" (48). This exchange takes an interesting turn when, for our benefit, the narrator adds, "I didn't know if what I was saying was true, I was not familiar really with immigration policies and HIV, but what I really meant was, no, I can't do what you are suggesting—take this strange, careless person into the hard-earned order of my life: my life of children and husband" (49). Crossing borders becomes a threat to the stability of Kincaid's marriage and her otherwise conventional domestic arrangement. In contrast to this "husband" who exists within a legally recognized framework, the border and the act of crossing it pose a threat to the state-sanctioned structure of Kincaid's nuclear family. When the news of her brother's illness "interrupted" (151) "the life with [her] own family" (151), she recalls, "I was in my house in Vermont, absorbed with the well-being of my children, absorbed with the well-being of my husband, absorbed with the well-being of myself" (7). In imagining her brother crossing national borders into her American family, Kincaid demonstrates a need to reinforce the impermeability of this nuclear unit. She emphatically asserts that "they love me and love me again, and I love them" (49). This persistent reassurance of love—repeated always in threes to mirror the nuclear trinity of self/husband/children—figures Kincaid's own migration as creating her American family in opposition to her brother, for whom she repeatedly asserts a "conflicted" (Stanton 45) lack of love: "I did not love him. What I felt might have been love, but I still, even now, would not call it so" (Kincaid, *My Brother* 58).

These assertions of the love and stability that the narrator finds in her American family but not in her Antiguan family again resurface whenever she discusses her brother in an explicitly sexual way. For instance, when Devon tells his sister about his teenage exploits with public sex, her narrative jarringly jumps from Antigua back to Vermont. While at one moment Kincaid is "walk[ing] back to my mother's house" (81), in the following paragraph, without any further explanation, she narrates, "I returned to my own home in Vermont with my children" (81). Through this non sequitur transition, Kincaid's narrator reasserts her caregiving role as belonging not with her "strange, careless" (49) brother in Antigua but with her nuclear unit in the United States. Because the narrator is able to separate her brother conceptually from her family, she cannot envision Devon crossing the borders into her own seemingly protected life. The narrator attempts to position the family and her responsibilities within it as requiring her continued migration away from her brother and his disability. Her sense of family thereby becomes bounded by American narratives of kinship as legally sanctioned and free of disease.

The narrator's discomfort with these diasporic kinships can further be read as connected to her uneasiness around bodies and their sexual representation. The narrator positions her brother's decision "to conduct his life so heedlessly" (29) against her own conservative sexual practices. She humorously discloses, "My own life, from a sexual standpoint, can be described as a monument to boring conventionality. And so because of this, I have a great interest in other people's personal lives. I wanted [my brother] to tell me what his personal life had been like. He would not do that" (41). These short, direct sentences—"he would not do that"—contrast the impressively long sentences that are connected to one another by semicolons rather than fully separated, and are used to describe the mounting tension between the narrator and her mother. While Kincaid's short sentences create a deceptive sense of narrative certainty, these long sentences indicate moments of unprocessed trauma, often cycling back to the same heated moment when the narrator neglects to change her brother's diapers when forced as a teenager to do child care instead of attending school:

> When my mother saw his unchanged diaper, it was the realization of this that released her fury toward me, a fury so fierce that I believed (and this was then, but even now many years later I am not convinced otherwise) that she wanted me dead, though not in a way that would lead to the complications of taking my actual existence and then its erasure, for she was my mother, my own real mother, and my erasure at her hands would have cost her something then; my erasure now, my absence now, my permanent absence now, my death now, before her own, would make her feel regal, triumphant that she had outlived all her inferiors: her inferiors are her offspring. (131)

This running sentence structure also indicates the narrator's failure to neatly resolve this event or to eventually come to terms with how the caregiving labor needed for her brothers actually erodes the connection between the narrator and her mother:

> But there was a moment when in a fury at me for not taking care of her mistakes (my brother with the lump of shit in his diapers, his father who was sick and could not properly support his family, who even when well had made a family that he could not properly support, her mistake in marrying a man so lacking, so lacking) she looked in every crevice of our yard, under our house, under my bed (for I did have such a thing, and this was unusual, that in our family, poor, lacking a tradition of individual privacy and whether this is a good thing, whether all human beings should aspire to such a thing, privacy, their thoughts known only to them, to be debated and mulled over only by them, I do not know), and in all those places she found my books, the things that had come between me and the smooth flow of her life, her many children that she could not support, that she and her husband (the man not my own father) could not support, and in this fury, which she was conscious of then but cannot now remember, but which to her regret I can, she gathered all the books of mine she could find, and placing them on her stone heap (the one on which she bleached out the stains and smudges that had, in the ordinariness of life, appeared on our white clothes), she doused them with kerosene (oil from the

kerosene lamp by the light of which I used to strain my eyes reading some of
the books that I was about to lose) and then set fire to them. (133–34)

The repetitive, elongated cadences through which the narrator emphasizes the
biological ties to and harms from "my mother, my own real mother" (131) contrast the sparseness with which she describes the distant relationship between
herself and her (half) brother who, as she claims, also hides parts of himself from
her. The assertive structure of "he would not do that," which ends the sentence
about "that" object of Devon's failed action, mirrors this long sentence's end, "and
then set fire to them," emphasizing the effect of caregiving burdens on "them"
and her mother's active success in destroying the narrator's educational (and as
we come to learn, sexual) opportunities, as symbolized by the burning of her
library. This narrative unearthing of family secrets, and of how nonconsensual
caregiving can threaten family bonds, is introduced as a theme that is both
emphasized and masked through these drastic differences in sentence lengths,
and by the omissions and returns to this memory and its representation that
transpire through gaps and jumps in the plot.

Despite these straightforward claims to her brother's secrecy, we actually
come to realize that not only does the narrator's brother frequently recount his
sexual experiences to his sister but she actually witnesses him flirting with, prop-
ositioning, and even dating multiple women. We also learn, at *My Brother*'s
conclusion, information we could have received far earlier in the narrative: Devon
also participates regularly in Antigua's private queer community. The narrator's
earlier assertion of her "great interest" in such matters is underwritten by her
constant reversion in these moments of disclosure back to the "boring conventionality" (41) of Vermont. The seemingly unmotivated jump cuts through the
story's space also indicate how the narrator's personal relationship to family and
identity cannot be rooted only in the United States or in the Caribbean, as her
narrative refuses to claim either location as mutually exclusive or as singly
"home." For instance, the narrator finds herself needing to clarify where she
means when she uses the term, "I was so happy to reach my home, that is, the
home I have now made for myself, the home of my adult life" (98). "Home" is
also always associated not with belonging but with loneliness, as the narrator
longs for her husband and children while visiting her brother in Antigua, and
she expresses sentiments of grief while "home" in Vermont. Like the distance
she keeps from her mother, her relationship to her father is also complicated, as
she continually reminds the reader (in brackets) that her father is not her biological father, and that he has always been closer to her than to his own biological children. When the narrator learns of his death in a letter, months after the
fact, she explains, "I had received the letter just before the Christmas season, and
it made a time when I was always unhappy even more so. I had many friends, but
they were not my family. I wept" (119). In representing the barriers to establishing

friends as chosen family while separated from biological family via migration, Kincaid complicates the stability of home that her narrator attempts to situate in Vermont. In identifying the disjuncture between the narrator's assertion of safety in home and Kincaid's undercutting of this possibility, the reader can begin to identify the futility of the narrator's desire to locate her own brother as existing apart from her (hetero-American) family.

These disconnects between the author and her persona accordingly undercut the narrator's attempts to place her brother as outside of her own sexual and nationally constructed norms. Through depictions of her brother's sexuality, the narrator repeatedly renders HIV as antithetical to her own legally sanctioned practices of monogamy and marriage. In Antigua, the narrator emphatically upholds heterosexual marriage as a safeguard against disability. Upon encountering one of her brother's old friends in the market, the narrator portrays him as an emblem of health because he appears in public with a woman and a child. She observes how "the three of them were together and they were a family and they looked so very nice, like a picture of a family, healthy and prosperous and attractive, and also safe" (112). HIV threatens the so-called safety not only of her own life in Vermont but also of the nuclear family itself. Because the narrative blurs generic borders between autobiography and biography, we come to understand Devon's queer desires only through his sister's textual re-creation of events. By spending the bulk of the narrative feigning a lack of knowledge about her brother's sexuality and withholding this information from her reader, the climactic moment of the story is not positioned with Devon's death (which happens halfway through the text at the start of the second of two parts) but with the reveal at the end of the book that Devon is queer.

The narrative timing of this outing is significant because in addition to the memoir's surprise all-along queerness, the big reveal also makes clear that our narrator quite intentionally selects what to share with us and what to hold back. Because the narrator's discovery of her brother's sexuality is sequestered to the narrative's end, this moment of disclosure undermines both the authority of this narrator as a reliable storyteller and her attempt to set borders around sexual, familial, or national identification. Rather than rehash the narrative of the doomed homosexual brother dying of AIDS, Kincaid instead underhandedly guides her reader to focus not on narratives of queer decline but on health-care access barriers that are created by colonialism and antiblack racism. Thwarting historically entrenched narratives that conflate nonnormative sexuality and disability with national decline (Marshall 24; Duncan 24; Showalter, *Sexual Anarchy* 4; Watney, "AIDS" 61; Snorton 4–5), Kincaid's memoir instead destabilizes these very identity categories through diasporic representations of caregiving. Through her narrator's inability to assimilate this information into the story without a climax, Kincaid herself challenges fixed understandings of nationality, disability, and sexuality, a project Juana Maria Rodriguez identifies as central to the generative work of HIV activism (34, 59). The narrator's disclosing of her brother's sexuality so late in the text actually writes his desires as fluid and as impossible to pin down, much like the diasporic space that prevents "home" from manifesting in only one location for his sister. In returning to this queer kinship model, early HIV caregiving literature provides an ongoing narrative framework for continuing to understand families, desires, and borders with the narrative openness though which Kincaid undercuts the attempted rigidity of her own narrator.

By bringing this early HIV narrative into the present, the kinships and migration patterns that form to provide care in spite of national borders continue to offer ongoing models for queer and trans disability movements in opposing the state violence of capitalism. Extending her observations of the postcolonial economy wherein "in Antigua itself, nothing is made" (Kincaid 24), the narrator continually repeats her brother's failures to "make something" (70): "I felt ashamed" (13), confesses the narrator, as she repeats again for the reader this same evidence of her brother's failures within a capitalist economy, his dying "without the traditional attachments to an ordinary man his age . . . a wife, a companion of some kind, children, his own house, even a house he rented, his own bed" (173). The narrator measures her brother's worth in his ability to give care, upholding his skills as a gardener, as the two share a love of caring for plants. In the final pages, the narrator again questions her own tears at her brother's funeral, wondering why she cried for someone who was a recipient but not a giver of care: "So many times we used to say that if by some miracle Devon could be cured of his disease he would not change his ways; he would not become industrious, holding three jobs at once to make ends meet; he would not become faithful to one woman or one man" (195). The narrator compares Devon with her other brother Dalma, worker of three jobs, who despite his capitalist ethic also remains living without his own family, in his mother's house, a narrative dismissed as "another big chapter" (81) rather than as evidence that links her brothers'—and national economic—dependency not to their individual failures but to ongoing histories of antiblack racism and colonization.

Kincaid offers a narrative critique by undercutting her own narrator's limited vision of kinship models themselves. This work connects early HIV caregiving to ongoing expansions of family in order to address medical injustice and disability into the present. The narrator depicts her family of origin in continued narrative opposition to colonial, individualist models of nuclear family. The narrator regards the creation of family as something that cannot coexist with living with one's mother. This is a narrative Devon himself plays into (perhaps for his sister's benefit) but does not act on. When Devon leaves the hospital, he tells his sister that he wishes to move out of his mother's house and start his own family (57). She assumes a straight, monogamous, nuclear family with biological kin, feeling pity that Devon can no longer heterosexually reproduce in nondisabled ways. As with her sexuality, the narrator's feelings about colonial trauma surface not directly but through her biographical musings on her brother. The trust we initially build with our narrator is called into question by the blame and judgment that she—but arguably not Kincaid—places on Devon for living with HIV. Although her narrator continually asserts that Devon's illness is his "own fault" (49), Kincaid shows the reader how ongoing histories of colonialism create multiple access barriers to Devon's care. For instance, while the leader of workshops remembered at customs attributes Devon's experience to "racism" (49), the narrator emphatically refutes this possibility, insisting instead that Devon's health-care barriers are instated by "the sheer accident of life . . . his not caring about himself . . . it was the fact that he lived in a place in which a government, made up of people with his own complexion, his own race, was corrupt and did not care whether he or other people like him lived or died" (49–50). In delving into why Devon is incapable of "caring about himself," the narrative repeatedly presents a gap between the narrator's assertions and those of the author (Stanton 51). The reader is then pitted between these two perspectives, one that links health-care access barriers to racism and to ongoing colonialism, and the other that renders these barriers to the "sheer accident of life" and to the "fault" (Kincaid 49) of Devon.

Reading this gap between narrator and author challenges national storytelling about HIV and about sexual norms, thereby underwriting the narrator's judgment of her brother. Kincaid thus offers a queer narrative of family for ongoing caregiving models of disability kinship in response to state violence. While the narrator attributes her disconnection from her brother to his secrecy, his homosexuality, and his illness, Kincaid presents us with the contradictory evidence of Devon's forthcoming nature, his sexual openness, and his playful critique of his sister's assimilation into colonial culture: "he would speak to me with a pretend English accent" (56). The narrator, in spite of all she learns about her brother as he is dying, laments not really knowing her brother at all. She then rereads her earlier analysis of his sexual confidence as erroneous. She reassesses his sexual advances toward women as a performance intended to hide his true desires, the expression of which she understands only through his outing by a white American lesbian. This woman tells the narrator in Chicago, after Devon's death, of the private queer event she organizes in her home in Antigua out of sympathy for "the homosexual man" (161), whom this white woman understands as having "no place to go" (161). Transnational queer theory warns against this narrative trend to view the United States as sympathetic and elsewhere as homophobic (Puar, *Terrorist* xi). As Thomas Glave cautions, such discussions of queer identities within the Caribbean should not be conducted without a transnational analysis of how colonialism and homonormative violence operate to create such narratives (4–5). Puar argues that such narratives of homophobia within the global south establish local homonormative practices of queer assimilation, inspiring a return to the respectability values of Kincaid's Vermont (*Terrorist* xii). Puar identifies how queer identity formations in the United States are deployed imperialistically within transnational contexts in order to gloss over "its own policing of the boundaries of acceptable gender, racial, and class formations" (9). In their discussion of the rise of queer assimilationist politics, Lee and Motta assert that the responsibility for this shift is intergenerational. They lament, "We continue to live in a world that would like to see queer people dead (queer immigrants, imprisoned African American trans people, sex workers and other 'others') yet mainstream activism is distinctly focused on issues of 'inclusion' (military service, marriage equality)." Kincaid's unreliable narrator can therefore be read as a literary mechanism for extending early HIV activism to younger generations toward the goal of moving the locus of caregiving accountability back into U.S. borders: Kincaid's work—despite and because of her narrator's discomforts—challenges this homonormative storyline that homophobic, normalizing practices are located only elsewhere (Puar, *Terrorist* xi–xii; Corber 111; Garvey 95; Chowdhury 9).

This early HIV narrative thus offers an ongoing model for linking disability kinships to the larger ongoing narrative project of redirecting accountability back into American policing of black, indigenous, racialized, and disabled bodies. HIV caregiving in Kincaid's narrative offers a model for reframing disability as creating kinships toward the decriminalization of bodies that do not conform. In rejecting racist narratives of the United States as the epicenter of queer liberation, this outing moment with the white American woman in the Chicago bookstore can be reinterpreted. Akash Nikolas, for instance, understands the information given about the narrator's traumatic past as examples of queer trauma, "queer experiences of being thrown out by one's parents, being bullied in school, and being in the closet. Thus queer shame is all over Kincaid's texts" (71). Nikolas, accordingly, reads the gap between the narrator's and Kincaid's perspectives as the site of queer storytelling. Nikolas revisits Kincaid's interactions with the white American woman in the bookstore through this coding of the narrator's own queer desire as expressed through her brother's (Nikolas 71; Rahim 12). Nikolas regards Kincaid's flustered reaction to the woman's queer appearance as one of shared identification, and Kincaid's depiction of her whiteness as locating whiteness as American but queerness as rooted back in the Caribbean (69). Nikolas's reading thus shifts the locus of scrutiny away from the Caribbean and onto the reader, pondering how "perhaps the tendency to overlook queerness in Kincaid's texts is because critics find both author and narrator difficult. Who can close-read when you cannot get too close?" (70). This question of distance versus intimacy in *My Brother* can be regarded as a narrative tactic that urges readers to disconnect from personal identification with the narrator to consider instead the interplay of structural barriers on the characters' experiences and sexual expressions. In *Caribbean Pleasure Industry: Tourism,*

Sexuality, and AIDS in the Dominican Republic, Mark Padilla argues that the structural inequalities illuminated by HIV reflect ongoing colonial processes that create economies based on pleasure and exploitation (170–71). Padilla discusses how sex work brings together heterosexually identified married men in the Caribbean and gay-identified tourists, breaking down the homo/hetero binary as well as the spatial remove between these two locations (180): "Increasingly, what it means to be gay in places like the United States is intimately related to what it means to be gay—or, perhaps more intriguingly, what it means to be straight—in places like the Caribbean" (212). In imagining through Devon "what it means to be gay," Kincaid uses auto/biography to challenge these colonial constructions of pleasure and labor from within an exploitative neoliberal economy. The contact between Kincaid and the queer white woman becomes the novel's climax, not merely in outing Devon but in outing homonationalist narratives that shape ongoing cultural understandings of why bodies are privileged to or denied access to caregiving, to queer kinships, and relatedly, to pleasure (Morgensen 2).

This moment thus connects the barriers to caring for Devon to those of forming queer kinships between brother and sister in response to HIV. The narrator's understanding of queer male culture in Antigua as invisible and as shameful is also filtered through this white woman's testimony from Chicago, in spite of the narrator's own earlier observation that "Antiguans are not particularly homophobic" (Kincaid 40). In discussing homophobia in Antigua, the narrator explains that fear of difference is not linked to sexuality or gender per se but to the cultural trend to "disparage anyone or anything that is different from whom or what they think of as normal" (40). Not only is the narrator's understanding of her brother's disabled body one of pity, but she also imagines Devon's experience of crossing heterosexual norms as something full of "scorn" (162), "secrets" (176), and "shadows" (176). She therefore imagines Devon relating to men without the comfort and openness he uses when flirting with women. The narrator links Devon's inability within Antigua to "live with all of it openly" (162) to her own need to leave home and family to "become myself" (162). The potential alternate reading that Devon feels the same ease privately with men as he performs publicly with women—and that his sexuality operates fluidly and without shame between people of different genders without even prompting a need to "come out"—does not occur as a possibility to our now-American narrator. The narrator instead regards her brother as embodying multiple coexisting lives, each of which corresponds to the fragments through which she is able to remember her brother from across the ocean. She recalls a photograph of her brother that "shows a young man, beautiful and perfect" (92–93), which she describes as a counterweight to his "unspeakable" (93) behavior during that period, a time she separates from other facets of his life: his youthful achievements, his time in prison, his illness, his overt love of women, his unannounced—or at least unannounced to her—love of men: "I did not know which Devon she meant. . . . Which Devon was he" (190–91). Although the narrator, removed physically and emotionally from her home in Antigua, is unable to reconcile these various experiences of Devon's, Kincaid nevertheless frames Devon's seemingly inassimilable personas as interconnected through the harm and resilience created by access barriers, borders, and the ongoing impact of slavery and colonization. The narrator's irreconcilable memories of Devon in the moments she is able to visit him offer a parallel to the fragmented chronology of his caregiving that we receive in place of a linear sequence of events. The gap between Kincaid and the narrator again implies that the sister's understanding of her brother as shameful is only one possible interpretation, one shaped by the limits of forced migration as a barrier to queer kin becoming able to share ongoing intimacies, and the mutual exchange of care across diaspora space. This sibling disconnect is one Christina Sharpe identifies as reflective of "the precarities of the ongoing disaster of the ruptures of chattel slavery" (5). Sharpe identifies "the power of and in sitting with someone as they die, the important work of sitting (together) . . . we insist Black being into the wake" (10–11). Returning to this text thus positions HIV caregiving as a form of resistance to the institutional barriers and narratives set in place to prevent disability kinships.

I Did Not Take Care of Him

This next section looks specifically to representations of HIV caregiving within *My Brother* to offer an ongoing critique of colonialism and antiblack racism. I consider how forced migration prevents the narrator and her brother from forming queer kinships for mutual care. Kincaid's memoir thus narrates access to disability caregiving as a form of body sovereignty. Not only does our narrator withhold information about Devon's sexuality, but the narrative initially presents only bits and pieces of information about care. Kincaid's narrator resists positioning herself as her brother's caregiver, informing us, "I did not take care of him, I only visited him and took him medicines, his mother took care of him" (116–17). Just as the reader must wait to learn about Devon's queerness, the centrality of caregiving as a kinship tie between the narrator and her brother can only be understood via plot information that is concealed until the story's end. The narrator's only childhood memories of this brother are of caring for him: "When he was a baby, I used to change his diapers, I would give him a bath" (21). Switching from the past tense of the diaper change to the prospective giving of a bath, the narrator immediately shuttles us back into the present to talk about how she begins bringing Devon various forms of medication that are unavailable in Antigua (21). This act saves her brother from dying of AIDS in the hospital in which she visits him as an adult. The narrator recounts, "I felt happy, I felt pleased with myself, I even felt proud of myself. I had been instrumental in this" (47). Despite her "instrumental" labor in supporting Devon's treatment access, the narrator refuses to define her role as one of giving care. In another instance, the narrator recounts witnessing the hospital staff's serophobia, noting how others staying on her brother's hospital floor who were not living with HIV "were not treated with the aloofness, at-arms-lengthness, that was extended to my brother" (46). We can again infer from this statement that the physical and emotional intimacy that transpires between sister and brother transcends the "arms-length" forms of care that Devon receives from hospital staff. The narrator's unwillingness to identify herself as a caregiver is challenged by Kincaid's representations of these "instrumental" forms of intimacy for the reader. Although not acknowledged by the narrator herself, these acts of care bring brother and sister together across national borders, bridging the distance put onto their family because the narrator was forced to leave home as a teenager in order to work in the United States. The narrator's inability to name this caregiving labor connects her displacement from her family to her nevertheless persisting "instrumental" role in returning home in response to her brother's needs.

The kinds of intimacy established through care make it difficult for the narrator to identify as a caregiver, because of the emotional and geographic distance she experiences from her family. For instance, in recounting these hospital visits, the narrator also depicts her labor in finding an HIV medical specialist in Antigua and arranging to have him visit her brother. She is surprised that this doctor examines Devon warmly and kindly, chatting, bonding, laughing, and even touching him "with his bare hands" (33). This skin-to-skin contact stands in contrast with the behavior of Devon's friends who will not enter his room. While this distance the friends keep from Devon is framed initially as serophobia, it also triggers memories of our narrator's own childhood isolation: "We are not an instinctively empathetic people; a circle of friends who love and support each other is not something I can recall from my childhood" (42). Despite her "extraordinary memory" (75) upon which she prides herself, the narrator cannot recall her own experience of the kinds of family intimacy that Devon and her other brother, Dalma, share, relaying Dalma's words from Devon's funeral of "how close they had been when they were schoolboys together" (194); the narrator feels continually apart from her family, who have all nicknamed one another but not her. The narrator relays how Devon calls out each nickname as his dying words but omits his sister from this (childhood and adulthood) act of naming:

> He did not know who I was, and I can see that in the effort of dying, to make sense of me and all that had happened to me between the years he was three and thirty was not only beyond him but also of no particular interest to him. And that feeling of his lack of interest in me, his sister, of not being included in the roll call of his family, seemingly forgotten by him in the long

hours before he left the world, seems so natural, so perfect; he was so right!
I had never been a part of the tapestry, so to speak, of Patches, Styles, and
Muds. (175)

This traumatic experience of forced migration and "all that had happened to me"
also motivates the narrator's desire to "think of my brothers as my mother's
children" (21) and as "these small children who were not mine" (128) rather than
as her own siblings. She continually (and convolutedly) depicts her brothers in
relationship to each other and to their birth order rather than simply using their
names. As with the NAMES quilt and with Rebecca Brown's *The Gifts of the Body*
(discussed in chapter 4) where the process of naming acknowledges the impact
of AIDS loss on larger communities, *My Brother* also frames the process of naming as a family-based memorial act. But rather than keeping the family together,
the narrator's impressive memory becomes a source of family shame: "As I grew
up, my mother came to hate this about me, because I would remember things
that she wanted everybody to forget" (75). The narrator grapples with the problem of remembering "the moment [my mother] turned on me" (75). This incident of trauma when the narrator's mother burns her books continually surfaces
and is discussed indirectly (Rice 26); however, we do not receive the actual details
of this event—an event that links the narrator to her brother via caregiving—
until 130 pages into the 200-page book.

As the narrative progresses, we come to learn that the narrator's relationship
with her mother collapsed because the narrator failed to adequately care for
Devon while he was a toddler and the narrator was a teenager. The narrator
regards Devon's birth as a "family disaster" (151) that disrupted "the routine of
our life" (4), and "plunged our family into financial despair" (141), a crisis for
which she blames her mother, who "could not properly support the family they
had made" (128). The narrator also regards her brother's birth as the catalyst for
her mother's removing her from school for "no real reason" (74); this act of economic necessity prevents the narrator from writing her university entrance
exams. The narrator remembers her disdain for being kept home from school to
watch her brother: "I liked reading a book much more than I liked looking after
him (and even now I like reading a book more than I like looking after my own
children, but looking after my own children is something I cannot describe in
terms of liking or anything else), and even then I would have said that I loved
books but did not love him at all, only that I loved him because I was supposed
to and what else could I do" (129). This refrain of "what else could I do" is repeated
many times by the narrator's mother while Devon is dying: "'What to do,' which
by that time perhaps everyone in my family (the family I could not help having)
said as almost a constant refrain, 'What to do'" (151). The narrator links the catas-
trophe of Devon's death to that of his birth, when the family "I could not help
having" also did not know "what to do" to "support his added presence . . . and

I was sent away to support a family disaster I did not create" (150). In answering these dilemmas of "what to do, what to do?" (151), the links between the narrator's "family disaster" (blamed on her mother) and the ongoing colonialism causing poverty in Antigua (blamed on Antigua) become increasingly clear, as Kincaid places under scrutiny the narrator's insistence that her life experiences are individual rather than structural problems. While the narrator blames her mother for burning her books, Kincaid undercuts her own narrator's analysis of poverty by connecting these family breakdowns in caregiving to the racism and colonialism that affects individual lives.

This gap between the narrator's individual laying of blame and the author's critique of the structural violence that affects individuals is again illuminated through the depiction of care. The narrator likens her brother's need for care while dying to the care he needs as a baby, when instead of changing his diapers the teenage narrator reads novels and ignores him. Rather than calling him Devon to distinguish him from her other brothers, she continually reasserts her relationship to him via blood ("my brother"), moving across the tenses of his process of his dying (and of his living) to discuss his care: "My brother, the one who was dying, who has died, who while dying could not take himself to the bathroom and freely control his bowel movements, then as a little boy, two years old, wore diapers and needed to have someone change them from time to time when they grew soiled" (130). The narrator and her family are unable to "properly support" (129) Devon as a child, and further, the narrator and her family are unable to provide Devon with the care he needs as an adult: "'What to do,' and we did some things. But none of them prevented him from dying" (151). The narrator's earlier statement, "I did not take care of him" (116), recalls the convergence of her adolescent trauma in becoming her brother's caregiver, her adult failure to prevent her brother's death, and her inability as a teenager to remain living with her family in Antigua. The narrative exposes how national narratives in "a place like Antigua, with its history of subjugation, leaving in its wake humiliation and inferiority" (186), liken those who are living with HIV to children, "the definitio[n] of vulnerability and powerlessness" (32). Such disability narratives mark those in need of care as undeserving of local and transnational resource access.

A close reading of this text thus reveals how Kincaid—in opposition to the claims of her own narrator—exposes how caregiving for her brother both in the present and in childhood fails not because of the individuals in her narrative but because of colonialism. Racism and colonialism prevent the siblings from building a queer kinship by growing up—or "sideways" (Bond Stockton 11)—together, as the narrator also connects this adolescent moment of failing to care for her brother as terminating her own process of adolescent sexual self-discovery. Barriers to caregiving demonstrate the rupture in her family structure that blocks her brother's treatment access and her family's access to one another. In *The Republic of Therapy: Triage and Sovereignty in West Africa's Time of AIDS*, Vinh-Kim Nguyen discusses the concept of triage, wherein global initiatives addressing HIV decide which lives are worthy of treatment. Sovereignty, the power to determine who can assert power over life, and the decision not just to conquer and/or kill but to let people live (Nguyen 13), remains a structuring force in social relations postcolonially (Nguyen 114), as the corresponding desire to categorize, classify, diagnose, group, and "empower" is a holdover of practices from colonialism (Nguyen 133). Puar links this type of queer biopower to HIV, arguing how neocolonial necropolitics influence narratives of the state-supported right to live or to die (32–33; Rose 248). This process of triage becomes directly connected to storytelling and narrative; those seen as engaging in practices of "truth-telling" (Nguyen 10), of speaking openly and unprudishly about their serostatus and sexualities, are granted technical and bureaucratic access to care (Nguyen 12). Furthermore, people living with HIV are often designated for saving in contrast to those suffering from a host of other common and treatable diseases who are left to die (Nguyen 181). Nguyen thus regards increasing healthcare access as a project not merely about finding an end to HIV but also to the ongoing colonial practices of triage that act as barriers to universal care (183; Ghosh 72). While the narrator judges her brother for his "carelessness with his own life" (Kincaid 195) and for rejecting the "boring conventionality" that prevents disability, she later feels how his death affects her: "[It] suddenly made me sad, suddenly made me wish that this, my brother dying, had not happened, that I had never become involved with the people I am from again, and that I only wanted to be happy and happy and happy again, with all the emptiness and meaninglessness that such a state would entail" (102–3). Again pointing to her untrustworthiness, the narrator undercuts her own upholding of family borders, framing Devon's disability as opportunity to retrace ties with kin in Antigua and to cross her own sexual borders in writing about Devon's decision "to live so much without caution" (29). Despite her assertions that she is unable to love her brother and that "nothing good could ever come of his being so ill" (21), she finds that disability, while the source of loss, also generates care: "I wanted to thank him for making me realize that I loved him" (21). The narrator also recognizes the life-sustaining potential of disability in creating narrative, as she also depicts writing as self-care: "When I was young, younger than I am now, I started to write about my own life and I came to see that this act saved my life. When I heard about my brother's illness and his dying, I knew, instinctively, that to understand it, or to make an attempt at understanding his dying, and not to die with him, I would write about it" (196). Through a combination of withholding and revealing, deflecting and exposing, the reader is positioned as witness to this act to self-care (Mitchell 113). The reader is also presented with an illness narrative that strives to represent HIV not to stigmatize disability but "to bring up the fact that all of us face impending death" (Kincaid 101–2). Lorna Down argues that these narrative layers in *My Brother* unfix the meanings of HIV in Kincaid's factual/fictional representation of illness (20–21). In ending *My Brother* with this reflection on the narrative process, Kincaid makes explicit the narrator's self-conscious relationship to her imagined readers and their predetermined understandings of the genre.

Close-reading Kincaid's auto/biography ultimately reveals its fluidness within the borders of literary genres. In blurring generic and sexual borders through the narrator's unreliable depictions of caring (and of being unable to care) for her brother, Kincaid also presents the geographical positioning of HIV as addressing breakdowns in care that cannot be confined to a single locale (Chambers 113; Davidson 122; L. Bernard 123). Caregiving literature points to the arbitrary and flexible nature of borders themselves, complicating distinctions between "illness and health, perceived illness and health, and death and life" (Pearl, *AIDS Literature* 83). Through its representation of HIV caregiving and its failures, Kincaid's narrative destigmatizes disability by representing the queer kinships fractured and retraced in spite of and in reaction to forced migration. This text thus offers a literary model that links early HIV caregiving to ongoing disability kinships that shift criminalizing narratives of blame away from the individual and back onto the state.

THE DIRTY LAUNDRY OF THE PRISON SYSTEM

This next section moves from an investigation of *My Brother* to an analysis of HIV prison narratives to model ongoing disability kinships in response to state violence. Just as narrative becomes a tool with which Kincaid undercuts her narrator's faulting of Devon for his illness, narratives of early HIV caregiving in prisons support decriminalization and body self-determination into the present. As in *My Brother*, prison narratives of HIV caregiving reframe disability as a structural rather than individual problem. While the policing of borders relies on narratives of protection, the violent maintenance of prisons is connected to a narrative process that justifies separation rather than community-based forms of accountability. Much scholarship has already demonstrated that prisons increase rather than decrease harm (sachse 203; Spade 156; Ritchie, *Arrested Justice* 4; Ben-Moshe et al. 14). Existing research also identifies the disproportionate rates of HIV and HCV (hepatitis C) infection, insufficient medical treatment of HIV, and the plethora of other health-care access barriers that are created by prisons (Shabazz 234; Ware et al. 170–74; Geary 81, 86–87). Criminalization, as has been well documented, is experienced unequally by black, indigenous, and racialized populations that face the highest rates of policing and incarceration (Alexander 2; Ritchie, *Arrested Justice* 3; Spade 93; Shabazz 229; Geary 24, 76; Hartman 108, 222; Hoppe 3). HIV criminalization laws also predominately affect black, indigenous, racialized, and other already targeted populations, and racialized people living with disabilities are also criminalized for transgressing body norms (Cheng, "How to Survive" 88; McClelland and Whitbread 85; Schulman, "Dear PosterVirus" 112; Leigh 35; Ben-Moshe et al. xi; sachse 202–3; Ware et al. 164; Clare, *Brilliant* 122; Snorton ix). In "Crippin' Jim Crow: Disability, Dis-Location, and the School-to-Prison Pipeline," Nirmala Erevelles argues "'becoming' black and 'becoming' disabled are not merely discursive events but are material constructs shaped by the political economy of educational opportunity and social segregation" (94). Such constructs also intersect with gender-based violence. The incarceration and mainstream media justification, for example, of CeCe McDonald for defending herself against an openly racist and transmisogynist attacker provide a public cultural instance of legislative and carceral systems that render the lives of black, indigenous, and racialized trans women as expendable (Hamel 2012; Broverman, "After"; Snornton 196). A variety of print-based and digital art supporting activist campaigns and the eventual release of McDonald—who continues to work as an activist for decarceration—attest to the utility not of prison reform but of replacing the prison system with more effective forms of harm reduction and disability justice (Ben-Moshe 263; Loyd et al. 14; Spade 157; Ritchie, *Arrested Justice* 11; Shabazz 230). I again represent early HIV caregiving and the kinships it forms to understand disability narratives as undermining the existence of prisons, supporting Rashad Shabazz's observation of how "de-incarceration is the most effective strategy to combat the AIDS crisis in Black America" (230). As Emily Hobson identifies in *Lavender and Red: Liberation and Solidarity in the Gay and Lesbian Left*, "proponents of a social action response to AIDS were turning ever greater attention to criminalization and poverty. Indeed, organizing to confront HIV/AIDS in prisons would grow through the early 1990s and inform the prison abolition movement" (183). Caregiving narratives of HIV prison organizing thus catalyze present and future imaginings of prison abolition (Bell et al. 444).

Just as Kincaid's narrative offers ongoing literary tactics for decriminalizing migration, archives of early HIV caregiving activism can continue to inspire alternatives to police and prisons. The early HIV caregiving work of prisoners including the collective of ACE offers ongoing models for creating communities in response to disability, practicing forms of justice outside of the carceral system (Ben-Moshe 268). Returning to early HIV archives of caregiving also reframes antiprison work as a central component of disability activism. Early HIV archives represent caregiving alliances between HIV communities inside and outside of prisons, breaking isolation through improving (and documenting) access to care (PWA Coalition; Cheairs et al. 26). Eric Slade and Mic Sweney's 1992 activist video *Acting Up for Prisoners* follows the ACT UP/Los Angeles campaign to support the women living with HIV at Frontera prison in California. Introducing viewers to the "dirty laundry" of the prison system, this video presents a series of talking head interviews and ACT UP demonstration footage to address the

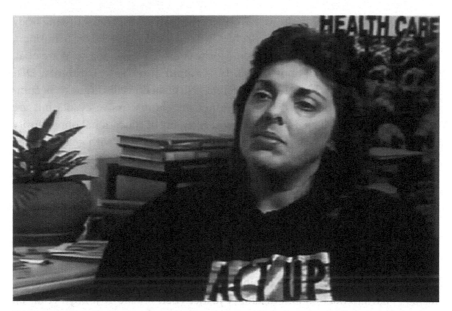

Figure 5.2. A still of Mary Lucey in Eric Slade and Mic Sweney's *Acting Up for Prisoners* (1992). Printed with permission from Mary Lucey, Eric Slade, and Mic Sweney.

barriers to care faced by prisoners. In an interview for the film, ACT UP member and former inmate Mary Lucey describes conditions of "women being dead in their cells for three days, nurses not touching women, guards ignoring women's cries for help, women not getting . . . prophylactic[s]." (See fig. 5.2.) Lucey attests to the importance of coalitional organizing, including documentary filmmaking, between prisoners and community on the outside: "The thing about the prison issues that occurred to us is that the population is completely hidden from view from the public. Unless someone raises the issue from the outside, the prison people can treat their prisoners any way they want to and no one will know." In another interview, Crystal Mason of ACT UP/San Francisco and the SF AIDS Foundation characterizes the prison as "a holding tank for people of color," illustrating how "few people are rehabilitated through the prison system." *Acting Up for Prisoners* attempts to document these injustices using the narrative medium of video. In considering what can be represented on screen, a reading of this video raises further questions of who has access to telling prison stories. Responding to HIV, the camera follows ACT UP protesters into the administration's head office to reinforce their previously stated demands. As the protesters are arrested and the climactic scene fades, a treble voiceover reflects, "It's so infrequent that there is a culprit that you can identify. This was one of those times where someone was doing something very wrong and it was causing harm to people with AIDS and they were right there." Interestingly, the documentation of this standoff entails not gaining access to an actual prison but rather bringing the camera (and the protest) into a sterile office building: the demonstrators use such pressure tactics as covering an administrator's framed credentials and office furniture with ACT UP sticky Post-it notes. The success of this direct action against bureaucracy thus reroutes the success of the video project; the focus of the camera becomes not the prisoners or the prison but the administrative route through which the carceral system operates (Spade 11). This shift from the prison pictured at the documentary's opening to the office building of the documentary's close raises questions about the obstacles to representing community alongside prisoners: what is a prison documentary if the camera cannot enter the actual threshold of these institutions?

HIV archives thus also raise a problem of representation, of how to create caregiving communities within institutions whose central function is to punish their inhabitants through isolation. Alexandra Juhasz's analysis of HIV media reminds us that with the invention of lightweight, portable, and affordable videorecording equipment in the 1980s came the rise of documentary media production by and for people living with HIV (*AIDS TV* 34). Such technologies, however, have been and continue to be denied to prisoners, effectively banning already marginalized populations from representing their own experiences. Even today, with the proliferation of personal digital recording devices—and with the increase of video surveillance mechanisms forced upon prisoners by guards—access to technology for prisoners remains limited if not contraband, furthering this process of nonrepresentation (Strauss, "Physical"). Connecting these media obstacles past and present reveals how prisons create gaps in caregiving through these barriers to technology access. In an ACT UP Oral History Project interview, Catherine Gund, codirector with Debra Levine of early HIV prison documentaries including *I'm You, You're Me* (1993) and *The Katrina Haslip Memorial Tape* (1992), discusses her experience of building HIV community with the women inside:

> There were a group of women that . . . thought that we could bring additional information, additional to the minimal, information that was allowed into the prison in Bedford Hills. And we talked about working together to have the women in Bedford Hills, who were in an organization that already, they had established, called AIDS Counseling and Education—ACE—and to help them make a video about what they were doing. So the goal was to go in, teach them how to use the video camera, help them do it, take out their footage, get their edit decision list, their EDL, and cut a video. So that there'd be a video about AIDS on the inside and the organizing they were doing. And then at the same time, to be able to feed any informational gaps or needs that they had that we could help out with, because we were busy writing a Women and AIDS handbook, and we were doing a lot of research. (43–44)

After outlining the vision for this collaborative project, Gund recollects the over-whelming obstacles to video-based self-representation within the context of prison: "So we got the permissions to go in and meet with the women of ACE. We had to wait on bringing a video camera in. . . . We went in, and we had some workshops together. We did some workshops where we did some trainings and teaching; they still weren't allowing a video camera in. Long and short, they never allowed the video camera in. And by the time we had gone through all their red tape . . . they slowly decided we weren't even allowed to come in anymore. So it dissolved, in my memory, pretty quickly" (44). Like *Acting Up for Prisoners*, which documents prisoner resistance without actually entering prison, Gund's HIV archive narrates these barriers to outside and inside collaboration. Gund and Levine concede to this access barrier by filming the work of former prison-ers including those organizing with ACE and ACE OUT (a group for women liv-ing with HIV who have been released from prison), connecting the camera to those spaces it was ultimately never permitted to enter. These technological bans create a lack of accountability for human rights violations in prisons and give dominance to media narratives normalizing the substandard medical access that prisoners receive. As outlined by the Prisoners with HIV/AIDS Support Action Network (PASAN), a Toronto-based organization holistically addressing the overrepresentation in prison of HIV and HCV, prisoners are actually entitled to comprehensive medical care, despite the "direct or indirect barriers to access-ing health services in prisons" (14; Namaste 47). Denying prisoners access to technology thus becomes a barrier to self-representation, creating a phenome-non where experiences of prison life are filmed by those outside of prisons, silenc-ing the perspectives of those most marginalized. In addressing this narrative gap, returning to early HIV archives of prison caregiving offers a model for con-tinuing to disrupt the isolation of prisons.

AND WE JUST TRIED TO BE SUPPORTIVE TO ONE ANOTHER

This chapter concludes by revisiting the early HIV caregiving archives of Gund and Levine to offer ongoing disability kinship models for prison abolition. These now-archival narratives that remain in the New York Public Library's AIDS activist video collection commemorate the work of the HIV peer-support net-work, ACE. *The Katrina Haslip Memorial Tape* presents a series of interviews and activist footage in which Katrina Haslip depicts the work of ACE in creat-ing HIV communities in prison. Haslip, a Muslim HIV activist who identifies as straight, discusses the creation of ACE. In the video, Haslip clarifies that ACE was actually conceived in 1985, prior to her arrival at Bedford. Haslip explains how she became involved with ACE before she learned her own HIV status, emphasizing the role of care rather than serostatus in creating HIV community. Haslip depicts the climate that incited the collective formation of ACE through which women in prison began to organize formally in response to disability. She recalls that "the original core group was living with seeing people physically or verbally abused, seeing people isolated [. . . and] seeing people with AIDS' cells being burnt up. I think . . . that was beginning to get them to start talking about it: how do we change this? What role can we play in this?" (*Katrina Haslip Memorial Tape*). ACE offers a narrative model of care in addressing this question of what role to play in response to abuse. The publications of ACE discuss this history of human rights violations caused by HIV stigma: "In an Alabama prison, in the early period of the AIDS epidemic . . . a prisoner who was HIV-positive had to wear a gown, gloves, and mask, and spirt disinfectant over each step every time she left her cell" (Members of the ACE Program of the Bedford Hills Correctional Facility 202). Within a system that places queer, trans, and gender-nonconforming prisoners in solitary confinement for "their own protection" (Mogul et al. 93, 103), HIV has repeatedly been cited as justification for the further marginalization of those already facing violence in prison. Prisoners living with HIV are denied low-level-security classification, participation in early release programs, conjugal visits, and other rehabilitative programs that can be withheld from prisoners simply because they are living with HIV (Mogul et al. 98; Stockdill 137). Responding to narratives of disability stigma stemming from a lack of accurate knowledge about HIV transmission, the "core group" of ACE coalesced to address these intertwined issues of access to care and access to information. In the video, Haslip addresses this gap in knowledge, recalling how, at first, "[they] knew very little about AIDS" (*Katrina Haslip Memorial Tape*). In order for ACE to provide support and services, Haslip explains, "we knew that we would need education from outside resources . . . and we got that training, we got volunteers to come in from [the] hospital, from the department of health, from ACT UP, from HEAL, and they did an education process with us" (*Katrina Haslip Memorial Tape*). Haslip recollects the development of HIV caregiving work within a prison setting, observing how initially, this work took place in an unofficial capacity, operating on the level of day-to-day prison life: "We were doing counseling one-on-one—informally, in the yard, in the shower—you know, wherever people ask questions. And we just tried to be supportive to one another" (*Katrina Haslip Memorial Tape*). Haslip traces how functional spaces in prison—showers, recreational spaces, common areas, kitchens—create opportunities to discuss experiences with HIV, substance use, and sex. Haslip's narrative models how the informal daily intimacies and acts of support exchanged in response to disability can transform mundane everyday spaces of confinement into spaces of collective care (*Katrina Haslip Memorial Tape*).

In narrating the formation of ACE, Haslip explains how these daily forms of caregiving create connections between women who were intended to remain isolated from each other, as well as from their communities outside of prison. She observes, "We were strangers. We were these supposed 'criminals' . . . the

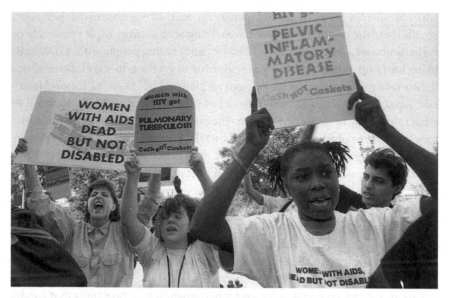

Figure 5.3. Photograph of ACE (AIDS Counseling and Education) collective member
Katrina Haslip. Photo by Donna Binder.

outcasts of society that [were] responding to the epidemic in a way that some
communities out here were not even responding, and that really made us hyped"
(*Katrina Haslip Memorial Tape*). In *Breaking the Walls of Silence*, a 1998 published volume documenting ACE's history and work, the collective of authors
from ACE also note how HIV organizing coalesced in spite of these conditions
of isolation: "We were building [ACE] from behind a wall, from prison. We were
the community that no one thought would help itself. Social outcasts because of
our crimes against society, in spite of what society inflicted against some of us"
(10). ACE points to the transformative role of "help itself" in preventing harm,
suggesting that had "what society inflicted" been met with support and not isolation, there would be no need to form a "community" of "outcasts" asserting
their rights to care: "We want something to happen, we refuse to remain silent;
we're not just going to go away" (*Katrina Haslip Memorial Tape*). (See fig. 5.3.)
Haslip asserts her own immovability and the success of ACE to contest narratives of expendability that justify the removal of "supposed 'criminals'" from
their communities.

These prison archives offer an ongoing model of kinship formations in
response to disability that counter criminalization and isolation by bringing
"strangers" together as caregivers. Returning to these early narratives of HIV
demonstrates the activist potential of caregiving in replacing the isolation of prisons with community-based forms of anticarceral justice. These daily supportive
acts in response to disability build HIV communities as a means of decreasing

harm and violence. As the collective of ACE elaborates, "We were inspired by the example of the gay community coming together to fight AIDS. From publications such as *The PWA Newsline* and *Surviving and Thriving with AIDS*, we learned about PWAs who were fighting to transcend their condition as victims" (Members of the ACE Program of the Bedford Hills Correctional Facility 25). Extending the gay communities of care that began outside of prisons, Haslip recalls the in-prison community formations supported by ACE: "We began to link PWAs (People with AIDS) up with buddies who would go up to the hospital to see them, who would do their shopping or clean up their cells, or help them in the shower, or take them out for recreation. And we noticed that it was really becoming something, it was changing the community. And we were seeing ourselves as a community, and we were very hyped about it because we were the community that was invisible, that no one thought could help themselves, and yet we were doing it" (*Katrina Haslip Memorial Tape*). Again, functional, daily acts like shopping, cleaning, and providing help with unpaid labor build community in response to disability. In creating conditions for "seeing ourselves as a community," the HIV caregiving of ACE also pressured the prison administration to acknowledge the impact of informal care as "changing the community." Haslip recounts, "As a result of all of that, the agencies noticed that we were responding, and they rewarded us a quarter of a million dollars to run a program for the staff and to set up office equipment and supplies that we really needed, and that's how we actually became ACE" (*Katrina Haslip Memorial Tape*). The shift from informal acts of breaking isolation to the institutionally supported provision of care indicates the power of prison administrations to encourage or to prevent the formation of communities in prisons; many of these HIV caregiving programs from the early 1990s have since been disbanded under "anti-gang" laws that prohibit in-prison community formations (Shabazz 235). Recalling ACE's narratives thus continues to respond to HIV as opportunity for collaborations and kinship formations, building communities across carceral spaces toward eliminating prisons. By re-centering decriminalization within narratives of disability activism, Haslip's words can continue to inspire younger generations of community caregivers to "always find a way to motivate ourselves. . . . We must find a way to use the smallest success as an incentive to keep on doing this work, and by all means, we must not allow prisoners to be invisible. Let's keep the pressure on" (*Katrina Haslip Memorial Tape*).

This chapter ends with ACE to return to where chapter 1 begins, reading narratives of HIV kinships as reframing disability not as a site of shame but as opportunity for decriminalization and decarceration. Kincaid's literary strategy of creating a gap between her narrator's persona and her own authorial voice offers an ongoing critique of colonialism that bridges early HIV caregiving with contemporary disability kinship formations. In resisting borders and familial displacement through auto/biography, I connect Kincaid's caregiving narrative to the prison caregiving narratives of *Acting Up for Prisoners* and of ACE toward *Forget Burial*'s broader goal of bringing early HIV archives into the present. This chapter thus surveys the diasporic, hospital, administrative, and everyday prison spaces in which care can be denied or exchanged. Like the previous chapters that bring together fictions and archives of chosen families and HIV communities in support of nonconforming bodies, these caregiving narratives offer queer and trans kinship models that imagine a future without police and prisons.

Conclusion

FORGET BURIAL

As I was finishing this manuscript and wondering how to conclude my decade of writing about a crisis that does not resolve, I was coming home to Toronto, and I saw a bumper sticker that has been appearing a lot lately: "Say No to Sex Education."[1] When I was a kid, my mom read aloud with me a bedtime book with a blue cover called *Say No to Drugs*, in which many different early 1980s cartoons that looked like the *Family Circus* presented various scenarios that prompted me to practice saying "No," apparently a widespread response (enough to win a provincial election) to our new (but soon to be disbanded) K–12 public school sex education curriculum that teaches kids beginning at age six about consent, queer-inclusive sexual expression, and trans-inclusive gender self-determination. By way of concluding this book, I want to end with what we as sex educators do when we say no to concluding early HIV narratives.

At the time of completing this manuscript, I have now shared this research in the form of sex education in college and university classrooms in all four cities I've lived in since I started writing: New York, Montreal, Atlanta, and Toronto, in that order. In each classroom, regardless of the school's and/or city's political leanings, I've had endless students who had never received any form of sex education, who were taught that it's sinful to even think about sex (including straight sex), who don't know the difference between HIV and AIDS, who don't know how HIV is transmitted, who have never heard of ACT UP, Iris De La Cruz, rimming, or pre-exposure prophylaxis (PrEP). Most recently, of the thirty-five students in my upper-year Toronto university classroom, only one student had heard of PrEP. While teaching a "Gender and Sexuality in Literary Studies" course in

---

1. Conservative Ontario politicians created campaign platforms (stickers, even) that appeal to a desire to remove the newly created sex ed curriculum from our provincial public school curriculum because it informs children about sexual consent, queer-inclusive sexual expression, and gender self-determination.

2010, I asked a room of seventy students at a progressive university in Montreal the question, "Does anyone here know who invented safer sex," and one of my students shot up a hand and very confidently answered, "Was it the Pope?"

When I give my students trans 101 workshops in each of these cities, multiple students get up and leave the room each time I say aloud the word "penis." I have been told annually by students in course evaluations and to my face why I shouldn't teach queer content, why trans people can't exist, why my class made them queer, why I changed how they understand disability, why I was the only person in their whole life who supported them through a disability diagnosis. I tell these students to "say no" sometimes and we have moving and complicated conversations about sexual consent. We hold honest discussions about risk, about why sexually transmitted infections (STIs) are stigmatized and criminalized. We exchange compelling reflections on Octavia Butler. I have shared the content of *Forget Burial* in some way or another with all of them, as I have with all my friends and lovers, with HIV community, with my parents, with my uncle while he died of cancer, with doctors and specialists who continue to misdiagnose me and misgender me and complicate my own understanding of my body. In working on this project with everyone around me, I have formed the kinds of disability kinships that this book anticipates. I also needed a great deal of care and used this work to better understand my own disappointment upon not always receiving it. I have defined my own experience of becoming disabled through unburying these histories, and I continue to allow early HIV activism to shape my own changing relationship to my queer and trans body and its norms.

I also draw on these early HIV narratives to understand my own experiences of loss. My hope is that early HIV narratives can also inspire an ongoing collective caregiving response to support trans women experiencing state and interpersonal violence, as Kai Cheng Thom urges: "It is our responsibility to change the stakes, to offer different options, to keep reaching out and sending the message that we will never stop trying, never stop caring, never stop loving" (46). I worked on part of this project with my research assistant Emma Deboncoeur, who recently died before I could see her again and talk to her about all the trans things she found at the Gay and Lesbian Historical Society and about what I thought about while writing about these materials for four years. I notice often that I still anticipate having these conversations with her when I'm next in the Bay Area.

In 2015, I collaborated on a panel connected to this project with my old friend from New York, Bryn Kelly. She presented work with me by Skype for a conference (she couldn't get over the Canadian border to be there in person), but I haven't seen her in person since I moved away from New York in 2008. I'll never see her again. She was the first person I met as an adult who talked openly about living with HIV. She once teased me because she thought I looked so much like the person I was dating at the time; she actually said to my face that she couldn't tell which of us was which. I'll never have a chance to ask her whether she wants to read this manuscript or whether she really meant that about me and my ex. In fact, I'll never have a chance to ask her anything. People say that AIDS deaths are over here, but I am still losing friends in my mid-thirties to serophobia in the age of PrEP. Bryn Kelly wrote the most beautiful fiction about PrEP.

Forget Burial returns to these legacies of early HIV kinships because they support ongoing sexual and gender self-determination within contemporary disability movements. The queer and trans connections that formed in response to HIV do not merely demand that we romanticize models of care that exist without the state, or that we settle for state-funded models rooted in the scarcity and unequal distribution of labor and resources within capitalism. As Jules Gill-Peterson reminds us, a return to medical archives can allow us to transform the queer and trans present by "dismantling the racialized, class-stratified structure of institutional U.S. medicine" (*Histories* 199). The early HIV archive continues to model how care can be something queer, trans, and mutually connective that supports our genders and sexualities precisely by also resisting criminalization, capitalism, racism, and colonial violence: HIV caregiving narratives teach ongoing disability movements to fight the very inequalities that block care access within the state, and to value our body differences toward resisting the state instead of trying to find a queer and trans place within it.

I'll never have a chance to "say no to sex education" because this is the work that I've done every day since I was twenty-three and I decided to write a term paper about vampires and HIV that I rewrote until I learned how these histories shape how I can exchange care as my work, in my writing, for fun, in general. Why I am still here on this sofa, self-isolating in COVID-19, disabled only since the last four years of writing this, now lying horizontally with four pillows and an ice pack and trying to conclude about caregiving while wishing someone was here to help me manage my own daily needs around mobility and pain. To exchange fluids like Butler's vampires and to continue to reanimate the early HIV archives possibilities for expanding care. I feel connected to all the people who have used disabilities as opportunities to create queer and trans intimacies with me. I feel touched that all along, this project has put me into caregiving and cross-generational mentorship connections with so many early HIV activists. I feel moved that these activists have cared to archive their work and the work of those they lost, so that I can keep unburying it. While I am still failing completely at ever understanding their experiences, at least now I'm finally realizing why that is so. Why I don't know what it's like in my thirties to lose so many lovers and friends and to watch my whole community get bashed and sick. Even though I've lost some and I've been bashed—but less—thanks to the caregiving work of the generations before me. In concluding this book, I hope that in response to governments and bumper stickers and COVID-19, we can continue to draw on early HIV caregiving to continue to use sex education to win our struggles for defunding the police, prison abolition, and the end of capitalism.

Forget Burial revisits the caregiving kinships formed in prisons, at hospitals, in doing dishes, by vampires, and on bedside tables to value disability for expanding our interdependence. "The cure for AIDS is kindness," reads a hand-sewn banner by Jessica Whitbread, reminding us that bodies that care for each other can collectively prevent disappearance. HIV archives attest to the ongoing impact of our HIV heroes, mentors, and ghosts, imagining new futures through our kinships with those who care for us, those we care for, and those we have lost.

Acknowledgments

This book is thanks to all the queers who hold me and care for me and inspire my writing. I want to thank my chosen family for giving me the care I needed to write this book. Thanks to everyone who has cared for my insomnia, leg injury, busted back, brain injury, and my mental health, and to everyone who has been vulnerable with me in letting me take care of you. All the beautiful forms of crip connection in my life are so important to this book, and I'm sorry I can't figure out a way to thank everyone by name who has changed the way I think about disability.

I am also thankful that my biological family has been so endlessly supportive of my dedication to this work. My parents, Elinor Bornstein and Richard Fink, have been reading this manuscript in various forms for over a decade ever since they broke the bound copy of my dissertation in half so they could both read it at the same time at my graduation. Thanks Mom and Dad.

I have also been cared for by so many different kinds of mentors since I began writing about HIV vampires in 2006. This research started as a dissertation at the CUNY Grad Center: I want to thank my dissertation advisor Robert-Reid Pharr for so many hours of conversation and laughter about books in your office. Thanks also to my dissertation committee members Steven Kruger, Barbara Webb, and Sarah Schulman for your brilliance and care throughout the most formative stages of this project. I reached out to Sarah Schulman (who was not then a professor at my school but a stranger) by email to ask her for a list of relevant HIV readings and she sent me her phone number and then met me in person in the East Village! It was a delight. Thanks also to everyone on my dissertation committee for making me cry after my orals so I can better understand how little I know about what it was like to lose so many friends and lovers in the 1980s and 1990s. Thank you for your generosity with my learning.

Thanks to everyone who mentored me at McGill, Concordia, and Georgia Tech. Thank you Allan Hepburn, Marcie Frank, Jesse Molesworth, Carrie Rentschler, Miranda Hickman, Elspeth Brown, Erin Silver, Patrick "Pato" Hebert, Ann Cvetkovich, Maxine Wolfe, Rebecca Garden, William Spurlin, Jim Hubbard, Debra Levine, Catherine Gund, Jean Carlomusto, David Oscar Harvey, Bishnupriya Gosh, Jes Battis, Mono Brown, and Lauren Jade Martin, for your input on various early iterations of this research. Thanks to Alex Juhasz for changing the way I understand mentorship and friendship and organizing. Working with you and reading your words has completely transformed me. Thanks to Julia Lesage and to the anonymous peer reviewers at *Jump Cut* for editing my earlier writing on HIV and disability—your feedback really helped me think through my ideas. Thanks to Joan Gordon, De Witt Douglas Kilgore, Ranu Samantrai, and all the anonymous peer reviewers at *Science Fiction Studies* and at *Callaloo* who reviewed and edited my work on *Fledgling.* An earlier version of chapter 1 first appeared in *Science Fiction Studies.*

Thanks to the reference librarians and volunteers who care for the archives that I visited and for helping me find my way through them. Thanks to everyone at the New York Public Library Manuscripts and Archives Division, the Center Archives, the Lesbian Herstory Archives, the University of Victoria Transgender Archives, the ArQuives, and the Schomburg Center for Research in Black Culture. Thanks to Steven Fullwood for your work and guidance in the Joseph Beam papers. Thanks to Kerri Flannigan for your fabulous research assistance and friend love in accessing UVic's archives for me. Thanks Sid Cunningham for connecting me with all the gender trouble makers. Thanks to Johnny Nawracaj, Trish Salah, Ted Kerr, Susan Stryker, Viviane Namaste, and Morgan M. Page for supporting me over the years to fill gaps in what I could never seem to find on my own. Thanks also to everyone who donated their art as images for this book: your art, activism, and legendary work is what inspired me to write this. Thanks to Tamara Ching, Allan Clear, Zoe Leonard, Mirha Soleil Ross, Adam Garnet Jones, Mic Sweney, Julian Talamantez Brolaski, Dona Binder, and Iris House. Thanks to Kia LaBeija, I'm so excited to have your portrait on the cover!

Thanks to everyone who read an earlier draft and talked through it with me in bed or on the couch or over the phone or over ice cream: thanks Cee Strauss, JJ Levine, Selena Ross, Aubrey Laufer, Jay Shea, Katie Hudson, Maggie Schreiner, Liam Michaud, Athena Thiessen, EJ Brooks, Sarah Butler, Alex McClelland, Morgan Sea, Vincent Chevalier, Mikiki, AJ Withers, Alex Barrett, Riki Yandt, Laura Horak, Kai Cheng Thom, Nora Strunk, and Quinn Miller. Thanks to Katie Jung for making me a Forget Burial denim jacket. Thanks to Cait McKinney, Morgan M. Page, and Zohar Weiman-Kelman for sitting down with the full draft of the manuscript and identifying all the problems I couldn't. Thanks to Oliver

Pickle for deeply copy editing this manuscript on two completely separate occasions. Thanks to Tali Cherniawsky for your extensive administrative labor, feedback, indexing, and care for so many drafts and edits and roadblocks and mysteries, and for your late-night emails. Thanks to Loree Erickson for your brilliant feedback on the draft and for all your activist work which not only changed my book but also makes me realize what collective care means and why it's so sexy. Thanks to Jessica Whitbread for all your inspiration and advice on the manuscript and for making this book so hot and fantastic: your art, your feedback, and the way you live in the world makes me better understand HIV kindness.

Thanks to my friends at AIDS Community Care Montreal and the Prisoner Correspondence Project for sharing your insights and experiences. Thanks also to all of the writers, activists, and artists who let me write about you and your legacies. I am deeply moved by the work that you do. Thanks to everyone at Visual AIDS and *Corpus* for the inspirational approaches to HIV and the care you give to art. Thanks to Nathan Lee for without my even asking, mailing me a copy of *Undetectable*; it arrived at a perfect moment.

Thanks to Bryn Kelly, whose friendship and writing on HIV were integral. I miss you, Bryn. Thanks to Emma Deboncoeur for your research assistance on this book and for the beauty you brought to your art and to my project and to my day-to-day experience of using the Internet. I miss you, Emma. Thanks to Robert for eating my cooking and for letting me make you art about how much you hated tofu—you are also remembered and missed.

Thanks to all my colleagues at Ryerson and to the Faculty of Communication and Design and the School of Professional Communication for the support for this project. Thanks also to all my students at Concordia, Dawson, Georgia Tech, UofT, and Ryerson for so many important conversations that animate my research and my writing process. This project is also thanks to the support of the Social Sciences and Humanities Research Council of Canada.

Thanks to Eli Bortz and to the (then anonymous) peer reviewers at Vanderbilt University Press, Jennifer Brier and Brett Stockdill, who patiently reviewed what had clearly been a dissertation and then explained very concretely what I needed to do to revise it for publication. Thanks to Sara Jo Cohen and Monica Pearl for your dedicated and thoughtful feedback from Temple University Press—I really value what you brought to this project with your extensive reviews and years of support. Finally, thanks to everyone at Rutgers University Press for all the care you put into publishing this book. Thanks to Jasper Chang and Vincent Nordhaus for your editorial work and support. Thanks to Ellen Lohman for such thorough and insightful copy editing. A most special thanks to Kim Guinta for your editorial work. Your enthusiasm for my writing was so acutely needed from the second we connected about the project and throughout the time during which you mentored over a decade of work into becoming a book. Thanks to the anonymous reviewer at Rutgers for so generously guiding me to restructure and revise the manuscript, you truly helped me see this project through to completion.

Finally, thank you to everyone who responded to HIV in the 1980s and 1990s for being heroes, mentors, and ghosts. This book is thanks to you.

(April 2020)

Works Cited

ACT UP Women's Caucus. PrEP media and public health discourse, with link. *Facebook*, 10 Dec. 2014, 12:22 P.M. www.facebook.com/ACT-UP-Womens-Caucus-292677117603857/. Accessed 18 Oct. 2017.

"AIDS and Minorities in Philadelphia: A Crisis Ignored." 1986 Annual Report. *Bebashi: Blacks Educating Blacks about Sexual Health Issues*. Joseph Beam Collection. Box 17, folder 2. *Schomburg Center for Research in Black Culture*, Archives Division, New York Public Library.

Alaimo, Stacey. "'Skin Dreaming': The Bodily Transgressions of Fielding Burke, Octavia Butler, and Linda Hogan." In *Ecofeminist Literary Criticism: Theory, Interpretation, Pedagogy*, ed. Greta Gaard and Patrick D. Murphy. Urbana: U of Illinois P, 1998. 123–38.

Aldarondo, Cecilia, Roger Hallas, Pablo Alvarez, Jim Hubbard, and Dredge Byung'chu Kang-Nguyễn, with an Introduction by Jih-Fei Cheng. "Dispatches from the Pasts/Memories of AIDS." In *AIDS and the Distribution of Crises*, ed. Jih-Fei Cheng, Alexandra Juhasz, and Nishant Shahani. Durham: Duke UP, 2020. 183–216.

Alexander, Michelle. *The New Jim Crow: Mass Incarceration in the Age of Colorblindness*. New York: New Press, 2012.

Almeida, Shana. Make Your Kindness Political. *Facebook*. 6 Apr., 2020, 8:35 A.M. https://www.facebook.com/shana.almeida.7. Accessed 22 Apr. 2020.

Anonymous Queers. *Wake Up Queers or We're All Through*. 1992. David B. Feinberg Papers, Manuscripts and Archives Division, New York Public Library, Astor, Lenox, and Tilden Foundations.

Arriola, Aimar. "Spectres of Iris De La Cruz." *We Who Feel Differently Journal* 3 (Fall 2014), ed. Tedd Kerr. wewhofeeldifferently.info/journal.php#Aimar.

Arsenault, Jordan. "Silence = Sex(e)." *PosterVirus*. 2012. *Tumblr*. postervirus.tumblr.com/post/35974194219/silence-sex-the-new-equation-by-jordan. Accessed 4 Sept. 2016.

Atkins, Robert. "Photographing AIDS." *AIDS: The Artists' Response* 4.1, Ohio State University, 1989. Gran Fury Collection, Manuscripts and Archives Division, New York Public Library, Astor, Lenox, and Tilden Foundations.

Auerbach, Nina. *Our Vampires, Ourselves*. Chicago: U of Chicago P, 1995.

Ayala, George. Foreword. *Corpus*, ed. Jamie Cortez, 1.1 (Summer 2003): v–x.

Bailey, Marlon M. "Black Gay Men's Sexual Health and the Means of Pleasure in the Age of AIDS." In *AIDS and the Distribution of Crises*, ed. Jih-Fei Cheng, Alexandra Juhasz, and Nishant Shahani. Durham: Duke UP, 2020. 217–35.

Ball, Bradley. *Diaries*. Bradley Ball Papers, Manuscripts and Archives Division, New York Public Library, Astor, Lenox, and Tilden Foundations.

Baril, Alexandre. "Transness as Debility: Rethinking Intersections between Trans and Disabled Embodiments." *Feminist Review* 111 (2015): 59–74.

Barnhardt, Kate. Interview by Sarah Schulman. *ACT UP Oral History Project*. Interview no. 052. 21 Mar. 2004. http://actuporalhistory.org/interviews/images/barnhart.pdf. Accessed 1 Feb. 2016.

Bauer, Amy. Interview by Sarah Schulman. *ACT UP Oral History Project*. Interview no. 048. 7 Mar. 2004. http://actuporalhistory.org/interviews/images/bauer.pdf. Accessed 18 Nov. 2013.

Bauer, Louise Birdsell, and Cynthia Cranford. "The Community Dimensions of Union Renewal: Racialized and Caring Relations in Personal Support Services." *Work, Employment and Society* 3.2 (2017): 302–18.

Baynton, Douglas. "Disability and the Justification of Inequality in American History." In *The New Disability History: American Perspectives*, ed. Paul K. Longmore and Lauri Umansky. New York: NYU P, 2001. 33–57.

Beam, Joseph. "Caring for Each Other." *Black/Out* 1 (Summer 1986): 9–11. *Schomburg Center for Research in Black Culture: Archives Division*. Box 14, folder 2. New York Public Library.

———. "Introduction: Leaving the Shadows Behind." In *In the Life*, ed. Joseph Beam. New York: Alyson, 1986. 13–19.

Bell, Chris. "Introducing White Disability Studies: A Modest Proposal." In *The Disability Studies Reader*, ed. Lennard J. Davis, 2nd ed. New York: Routledge, 2006. 275–82.

Bell, Jonathan, Darius Bost, Jennifer Brier, Julio Capó, Jih-Fei Cheng, Daniel M. Fox, Christina Hanhardt, Emily K. Hobson, and Dan Royles. "Interchange: HIV/AIDS and U.S. History." *Journal of American History* 104.2 (Sept. 2017): 431–60.

Bellwether, Mira Darling. *Fucking Trans Women: Vol. 0*, 2010. fuckingtranswomen.com.

———. "Mira Bellwether and 'Fucking Trans Women' Zine: The Autostraddle Interview." Interview by Kennedy Nadler. *Autostraddle*. 9 Aug. 2013. autostraddle.com/mira -bellwether-author-and-illustrator-of-fucking-trans-women-zine-the-autostraddle -interview/. Accessed 3 Mar. 2014.

———. "Mira's Mirror." *LiveJournal*, miraarim.livejournal.com/. Accessed 12 July 2013.

———. "Ofelia De Corazon & Miranda Bellwether: Sex Educators, Writers & Activists." Interview by Anya De Montigny. *The ((O)) Word*, 11 Apr. 2014. www.womensextalkradio .com/?page_id=84. Accessed 12 Dec. 2014.

Ben-Moshe, Liat. "Alternatives to (Disability) Incarceration." In *Disability Incarcerated: Imprisonment and Disability in the United States and Canada*, ed. Liat Ben-Moshe, Chris Chapman, and Allison C. Carey. New York: Macmillan, 2014. 255–72.

Bennett, Marti. "Enchanted Forest." In *Gulf Coast Transgender Community: An Outreach Organization* (June 1998): 8. Transgender Archives, University of Victoria. Victoria, British Columbia, Canada.

Berkowitz, Richard. *Stayin' Alive: The Invention of Safe Sex, A Personal History*. Boulder: Westview, 2008.

Berlant, Lauren. *Cruel Optimism*. Durham: Duke UP, 2011.

Bernard, Kim. Interview by Alexis Shotwell and Gary Kinsman. *AIDS Activist History Project*. 5 Aug. 2015. aidsactivisthistory.ca/interviews/nova-scotia-interviews/#Bernard. Accessed 3 Nov. 2017.

Bernard, Louise. "Countermemory and Return: Reclamation of the (Postmodern) Self in Jamaica Kincaid's *The Autobiography of My Mother* and *My Brother*." *MFS: Modern Fiction Studies* 48.1 (Spring 2002): 113–38.

Bersani, Leo. "Is the Rectum a Grave?" In *AIDS: Cultural Analysis Cultural Activism*, ed. Douglas Crimp. Cambridge: MIT P, 1988. 197–222.

Binnie, Imogen. *Nevada*. New York: Topside, 2013.

Black, Anthea, and Jessica Whitbread (with the HIV Howler Advisory). "Editorial." *The HIV Howler: Transmitting Art + Activism* 1.2 (25 July 2018): 3–4.

Blair, Jennifer. "The Glove of Shame and the Touch of Rebecca Brown's *The Gifts of the Body*." *GLQ: A Journal of Lesbian and Gay Studies* 11.4 (2005): 521–45.

Bordowitz, Gregg. *The AIDS Crisis Is Ridiculous*, ed. James Meyer. Cambridge: MIT P, 2004.

Boucher, L. M., Z. Marshall, A. Martin, K. Larose-Hébert, J. V. Flynn, C. Lalonde, D. Pineau, J. Bigelow, T. Rose, R. Chase, R. Boyd, M. Tyndall, and C. Kendall. "Expanding Conceptualizations of Harm Reduction: Results from a Qualitative Community-Based Participatory Research Study with People Who Inject Drugs." *Harm Reduction Journal* 14.18 (2017): 1–18.

Brandt, Allan M. *No Magic Bullet: A Social History of Venereal Disease in the United States since 1880*. New York: Oxford UP, 1985.

Bride, Kate. "'Remembering Well': Sexual Practice as a Practice of Remembering." *AIDS and Memory*. Special issue of *Drain*, with Amber Dean, ed. Ricky Varghese, 14.2 (2016). drainmag.com/remembering-well-sexual-practice-as-a-practice-of-remembering/. Accessed 10 July 2017.

Brier, Jennifer. *Infectious Ideas: U.S. Political Responses to the AIDS Crisis*. Chapel Hill: U of North Carolina P, 2009.

Brophy, Sarah. "Angels in Antigua: The Diasporic of Melancholy in Jamaica Kincaid's *My Brother*." *PMLA* 117.2 (Mar. 2002): 265–77.

———. *Witnessing AIDS: Writing, Testimony, and the Work of Mourning*. Toronto: U Toronto P, 2004.

Broverman, Neal. "After Horrific Fight Leaves Man Dead, Trans Woman CeCe McDonald Accepts Plea." *Advocate* 2 May 2012. www.advocate.com/crime/2012/05/02/accused -trans-woman-cece-mcdonald-accepts-second-degree-manslaughter-plea. Accessed 31 May 2012.

Brown, Rebecca. *The Dogs*. San Francisco: City Lights, 1998.

———. *The Evolution of Darkness and Other Stories*. London: Brilliance Books, 1984.

———. *The Gifts of the Body*. New York: Harper, 1994.

———. "A Good Man." In *Annie Oakley's Girl*. San Francisco: City Lights, 1993. 93–146.

———. "Rebecca Brown: The Byronic Woman." Interview by Matthew Stadler. *Lambda Book Report* 8.3 (Oct. 1999): 6–8.

———. *The Terrible Girls*. San Francsiso: City Lights, 2001.

Browne, Simone. *Dark Matters: On the Surveillance of Blackness*. Durham: Duke UP, 2015.

Bryan, Jed A. "Crying 'Wolf!': The Genesis of the AIDS Epidemic." In *Confronting AIDS through Literature*, ed. Judith Laurence Pastore. Urbana: U of Illinois P, 1993. 68–78.

Bryan-Wilson, Julia. "Art and Activism in the Age of AIDS." *AIDS/ART/WORK*, 30 May 2008, The Graduate Center of the City University of New York, CLAGS. Lecture.
———. *Fray: Art and Textile Politics*. Chicago: U Chicago P, 2017.
Butler, Octavia. "Bloodchild." In *Bloodchild and Other Stories*. New York: Seven Stories, 2005. 1–32.
———. *Clay's Ark*. New York: Warner, 1984.
———. *Dawn*. New York: Warner, 1987.
———. "The Evening and the Morning and the Night." In *Bloodchild and Other Stories*. New York: Seven Stories, 1996. 33–70.
———. *Fledgling*. New York: Seven Stories, 2005.
———. "An Interview with Octavia Butler." Interview by Charles H. Rowell. *Callaloo* 20.1 (Winter 1997): 47–66.
———. "An Interview with Octavia E. Butler." Interview by Randall Kenan. *Callaloo* 14.2 (Spring 1991): 495–504.
———. *Kindred*. Boston: Beacon, 1988.
C., Tammy. "Does Your Dress Cause You Stress?" *Trans-Port: A Peer Support Group for All Transgendered Individuals*, July 1995. Transgender Archives, University of Victoria. Victoria, British Columbia, Canada.
Califia, Patrick. "Gay Men, Lesbians, and Sex: Doing It Together." In *Public Sex: The Culture of Radical Sex*. San Francisco: Cleis, 2000. 191–98.
Callen, Michael. Interview. *GMHC Oral History Project*. Interview 00950-AB. 30 June 1988. AIDS Activist Videotape Collection, Manuscripts and Archives Division, New York Public Library, Astor, Lenox, and Tilden Foundations.
———. "Remarks of Michael Callen: Gay Pride Rally, June 25, 1988." *People with AIDS Coalition Newsline* July 1988. People with AIDS Coalition Records, 1987–1993. Manuscripts and Archives Division, New York Public Library. Astor, Lenox, and Tilden Foundations.
———. *Surviving AIDS*. New York: Harper, 1990.
———, ed. *Surviving and Thriving with AIDS*. New York: People with AIDS Coalition, 1987.
Carey, Allison C., Liat Ben-Moshe, and Chris Chapman. "Preface: An Overview of Disability Incarcerated." In *Disability Incarcerated: Imprisonment and Disability in the United States and Canada*, ed. Liat Ben-Moshe, Chris Chapman, and Allison C. Carey. New York: Palgrave Macmillan, 2014. ix–xiv.
Carlomusto, Jean. Interview by Sarah Schulman. *ACT UP Oral History Project*. Interview no. 05. 19 Dec. 2002. http://actuporalhistory.org/interviews/images/carlomusto.pdf Accessed 4 Nov. 2018.
———, dir. *Sex in an Epidemic*. Outcast Films, 2009.
Carlomusto, Jean, and Gregg Bordowitz, dirs. *Current Flow*. GMHC Safer Sex Shorts, 1989.
Carlomusto, Jean, Alexandra Juhasz, and Hugh Ryan, curators. *COMPULSIVE PRACTICE*. Visual AIDS- Day Without Art, 2016.
Carlomusto, Jean, and Every Ocean Hughes. "Radiant Spaces." *Corpus*, ed. Alexandra Juhasz, 4.1 (Spring 2006): 73–79.
Carroll, Tamar W. *Mobilizing New York: AIDS, Antipoverty, and Feminist Activism*. Chapel Hill: U of North Carolina P, 2015.
Castiglia, Christopher, and Christopher Reed. *If Memory Serves: Gay Men, AIDS, and then Promise of the Queer Past*. Minneapolis: U of Minnesota P, 2012.

Castillo, Debra A., and Maria Socorro Tabuenca Cordoba. *Border Women: Writing from La Frontera*. Minneapolis: U of Minnesota P, 2002.

Chambers, Ross. *Facing It: AIDS Diaries and the Death of the Author*. Ann Arbor: U of Michigan P, 1998.

———. "Text as Trading Place: Jamaica Kincaid's *My Brother*." In *Economies of Representation, 1790–2000: Colonialism and Commerce*, ed. Leigh Dale and Helen Gilbert. Aldershot, England; Ashgate, 2007. 107–22.

Charlesworth, Dacia. "Transmitters, Caregivers, and Flowerpots: Rhetorical Constructions of Women's Early Identities in the AIDS Pandemic." *Women's Studies in Communication* 26.1 (Spring 2003): 1–15. *Literature Resource Center*.

Chasin, C. J. Deluzio. "Making Sense in and of the Asexual Community: Navigating Relationships and Identities in a Context of Resistance." *Journal of Community & Applied Social Psychology* 25 (2015): 167–80.

Chávez, Karma. *Queer Migration Politics: Activist Rhetoric and Coalitional Possibilities*. Urbana: U of Illinois P, 2013.

Cheairs, Katherine, Alexandra Juhasz, Theodore (ted) Kerr, and Jawanza Williams, for What Would an HIV Doula Do? Collective. *Metanoia: Transformation through AIDS Archives and Activism*. New York: Self-published exhibit guide, 2019.

Chen, Mel. *Animacies: Biopolitics, Racial Mattering, and Queer Affect*. Durham: Duke UP, 2012.

Cheng, Jei-Feh. "AIDS, Women of Color Feminisms, Queer and Trans of Color Critiques, and the Crises of Knowledge Production." In *AIDS and the Distribution of Crises*, ed. Jih-Fei Cheng, Alexandra Juhasz, and Nishant Shahani. Durham: Duke UP, 2020. 76–92.

———. "How to Survive: AIDS and its Afterlives in Popular Media." *WSQ: Women's Studies Quarterly* 44.1–2 (Spring/Summer 2016): 73–92.

Chevalier, Vincent, and Ian Bradley-Perrin. "Your Nostalgia Is Killing Me." *PosterVirus*. 2014. *Tumblr*. http://postervirus.tumblr.com/post/67569099579/your-nostalgia-is-killing-me-vincent-chevalier. Accessed 25 Mar. 2015.

Chin, Timothy. "The Novels of Patricia Powell: Negotiating Gender and Sexuality across the Disjunctures of the Caribbean Diaspora." *Callaloo* 30.2 (Spring 2007): 533–45.

Ching, Tamara. "Breaking Barriers, Building Bridges: National Congress on the State of HIV/AIDS in Racial and Ethnic Communities." 15 Sept. 1994. GLBT Historical Society. Transcript. Tamara Ching Collection. San Francisco, California.

———. "Stranger in Paradise: Tamara Ching's Journey to the Gender Divide." *A. Magazine* 3.1 (1993): 85–86. Tamara Ching Collection. GLBT Historical Society. San Francisco, California.

Chowdhury, Elora Halim. "Violence Against Women: We Need a Transnational Analytic of Care." *Tikun Magazine* 29.1 (Winter 2014): 9–13.

Christensen, Kim. "How Do Women Live?" In *Women, AIDS, and Activism*, ed. The ACT UP/NY Women and AIDS Book Group. Boston: South End, 1990. 5–15.

———. "In Our Own Hands." *Outweek* (3 July 1989): 34. Lesbian Herstory Archives. Brooklyn, NY.

Clare, Eli. *Brilliant Imperfection: Grappling with Cure*. Durham: Duke UP, 2017.

———. *Exile and Pride: Disability, Queerness and Liberation*. Cambridge: South End, 1999.

Clear, Allan. Interview by Sarah Schulman. *ACT UP Oral History Project*. Interview no. 178. 1 Mar. 2015. http://actuporalhistory.org/interviews/images/clear.pdf. Accessed 20 Sept. 2017.

Cohen, Cathy J. *The Boundaries of Blackness: AIDS and the Breakdown of Black Politics.* Chicago: U of Chicago P, 1999.

Cohen, Ed, and Julie Livingston. "AIDS." *Social Text* 27.3 (2009): 40.

Corber, Robert J. "Nationalizing the Gay Body." *American Literary History* 15.1 (2003): 107–33.

Cortez, Jamie. Introduction. *Corpus*, ed. Jamie Cortez, 1.1 (Summer 2003): xi.

Crimp, Douglas. *Melancholia and Moralism: Essays on AIDS and Queer Politics.* Cambridge: MIT P, 2002.

Critical Resistance. *Abolition Now! Ten Years of Strategy and Struggle against the Prison Industrial Complex.* Oakland: AK Press, 2008.

Crow, Liz. "Including All of Our Lives: Renewing the Social Model of Disability." In *Exploring the Divide*, ed. Colin Barnes and Geoffrey Mercer. Leeds: Disability Press, 1996. 55–72.

Cvetkovich, Ann. *An Archive of Feelings: Trauma, Sexuality, and Lesbian Public Cultures.* Durham: Duke UP, 2003.

D'Adesky, Anne-Christine. *Moving Mountains: The Race to Treat Global AIDS.* London: Verso, 2004.

Davidson, Diana M. "Ghosting HIV/AIDS: Haunting Words and Apparitional Bodies in Michelle Cliff's 'Bodies of Water.'" In *Spectral America: Phantoms and the National Imagination*, ed. Jeffrey Andrew Weinstock. Madison: U of Wisconsin P, 2004. 221–43.

———. "Writing AIDS in Antigua: Tensions between Public and Private Activisms in Jamaica Kincaid's *My Brother*." *Journal of Commonwealth and Postcolonial Studies* 10.1 (2003): 121–44.

Davis, Angela Y. *Are Prisons Obsolete?* New York: Seven Stories, 2003.

Davis, Estelle. (Panel speaker). "We Can't Police Our Way Out of the Pandemic." Zoom Meeting, 28 Mar. 2020. https://youtu.be/AK9ioHaTu38?t=4355. Accessed 25 Apr. 2020.

De La Cruz, Iris. "AIDS Politics." *Outweek* 48 (30 May 1990): 36, 43. Lesbian Herstory Archives. Brooklyn, NY.

———. "The Great Sero-Positive Seder: Or, Pigging Out on Passover." *People with AIDS Coalition Newsline* (July 1990). People with AIDS Coalition Records, 1987–1993. Manuscripts and Archives Division, New York Public Library, Astor, Lenox, and Tilden Foundations.

———. Interview. *GMHC Oral History Project.* Interview 01032-A. AIDS Activist Videotape Collection. Manuscripts and Archives Division, New York Public Library, Astor, Lenox, and Tilden Foundations.

———. "Invasion of the Patients from Hell at New York University Hospital or How I Spent My Summer Vacation." In *Positive Women: Voices of Women Living with AIDS*, ed. Andrea Rudd and Darien Taylor. Toronto: Second Story, 1992.

———. "More Kool-AIDS (With Ice)." *People with AIDS Coalition Newsline* (May, June, July 1990, Jan., Feb. 1991). People with AIDS Coalition Records, 1987–1993. Manuscripts and Archives Division, New York Public Library, Astor, Lenox, and Tilden Foundations.

———. "Sex, Drugs, Rock n' Roll, and AIDS." In *Women, AIDS, and Activism*, ed. The ACT UP/NY Women and AIDS Book Group. Boston: South End, 1990. 130–34.

———. "We're All Fighting for Our Lives." *People with AIDS Coalition Newsline* (Mar. 1990). People with AIDS Coalition Records, 1987–1993. Manuscripts and Archives Division, New York Public Library, Astor, Lenox, and Tilden Foundations.

Dean, Tim. *Unlimited Intimacy: Reflections on the Subculture of Barebacking*. Chicago: U of Chicago P, 2009.

Delany, Samuel R. "The Gamble." *Corpus* 3.1 (2005): 140–69.

———. "The Tale of Plagues and Carnivals." In *Flight from Nevèrÿon*. Middletown: Wesleyan UP, 1994. 181–360.

———. *Times Square Red, Times Square Blue*. New York: NYU P, 1999.

DeLombard, Jeannine. "Who Cares? Lesbians as Caregivers." In *Dyke Life: A Celebration of Lesbian Experience*, ed. Karla Jay. New York: Basic, 1995. 344–52.

Denckla, Matthew. "Symposium Details Transgender Traits." *San Francisco Sentinel* 21 June 1995. GLBT Historical Society. San Francisco, CA.

Denenberg, Risa. "Lesbian AIDS Activists: What Are We Doing?" *Outweek* 17 (15 Oct. 1989): 30–31. Lesbian Herstory Archives. Brooklyn, NY.

———. "Treatment and Trials." In *Women, AIDS, and Activism*, ed. The ACT UP/NY Women and AIDS Book Group. Boston: South End, 1990. 69–80.

———. "Unique Aspects of HIV Infection in Women." In *Women, AIDS, and Activism*, ed. The ACT UP/NY Women and AIDS Book Group. Boston: South End, 1990. 31–44.

———. "What about Women?" *Outweek* 54 (11 July 1990): 44–45. Lesbian Herstory Archives. Brooklyn, NY.

———. "What the Numbers Mean." In *Women, AIDS, and Activism*, ed. The ACT UP/NY Women and AIDS Book Group. Boston: South End, 1990. 1–4.

Denneny, Michael. "AIDS Writing and the Creation of a Gay Culture." In *Confronting AIDS through Literature*, ed. Judith Laurence Pastore, Urbana: U of Illinois P, 1993. 36–54.

Derkatch, Colleen. *Bounding Biomedicine: Evidence and Rhetoric in the New Science of Alternative Medicine*. Chicago: U of Chicago Press, 2016.

———. "The Self-Generating Language of Wellness and Natural Health." *Rhetoric of Health & Medicine* 1.1–2 (2018): 132–60.

———. "'Wellness' as Incipient Illness: Dietary Supplements in a Biomedical Culture." *Present Tense* 2.2 (2012): 1–9.

DiAna, DiAna. *Curlers and Condoms: DiAna's Hair Ego*. New York: 1st Book Library, 2003.

———. "DiAna's Hair Ego: 2012–13 Concordia University Community Lecture Series on HIV/AIDS." YouTube recording. 22 Mar., 2013. Lecture. https://www.youtube.com/watch?v=Yrk_Bbon1MQ. Accessed 3 Apr. 2018.

Dobbs, Bill. "If I Die . . . Picture of David Wojnarowicz." *Corpus* 4.1 (Spring 2006): 80.

Dodd, Zoë. "Meet the Harm Reduction Worker Who Called Out Trudeau on the Opioid Crisis." Interview by Allison Tierney. *Vice* 25 Apr. 2017. www.vice.com/en_ca/article/ez3m5a/meet-the-harm-reduction-worker-who-called-out-trudeau-on-the-opioid-crisis. Accessed 30 Apr. 2017.

———. (Panel speaker). "We Can't Police Our Way Out of the Pandemic." Zoom Meeting, 28 Mar. 2020. https://youtu.be/j6s_FZu9F1s?t=292. Accessed 25 Apr. 2020.

Dodge, Harry, and Howard, Silas, dir. *By Hook or By Crook*. Steakhaus Productions, 2001.

Down, Lorna. "Stepping out of the Kumbla: Kincaid's AIDS Narrative, *My Brother*." *Caribbean Quarterly* 53.3 (Sept. 2007): 16–29.

Driskill, Qwo-Li. "Doubleweaving Two-Spirit Critiques: Building Alliances between Native and Queer Studies." *GLQ: A Journal of Lesbian and Gay Studies* 16.1–2 (2010): 69–92.

Dryden, OmiSoore. (Panel speaker). "We Can't Police Our Way Out of the Pandemic." Zoom Meeting, 28 Mar. 2020. https://youtu.be/AK9ioHaTu38?t=3447. Accessed 25 Apr. 2020.

Duke, Alison, dir. *Consent: HIV Non-Disclosure and Sexual Assault Law*. Canadian HIV/AIDS Legal Network, Goldelox Productions, 2015. www.consentfilm.org/.

Duncan, Derek. "Solemn Geographies: AIDS and the Contours of Autobiography." *Autobiographical Que(e)ries*, special issue of *a/b: Auto/Biography Studies* 15.1 (Summer 2000): 22–36.

Dyck, Isabel. "Women with Disabilities and Everyday Geographies." In *Putting Health into Place*, ed. Robin A. Kearns and Wilbert M. Gesler. Syracuse: Syracuse UP, 1998. 103–19.

Edelman, Elijah Adiv. "Beyond Resilience: Trans Coalitional Activism as Radical Self-Care." *Social Text* 38.1.142 (Mar. 2020): 109–30.

Edelman, Lee. *Homographesis: Essays in Gay Literary and Cultural Theory*. New York: Routledge, 1994.

———. *No Future: Queer Theory and the Death Drive*. Durham: Duke UP, 2004.

Edelson, Stuart. "AIDS Journals: 1989–1992." Stuart Edelson Papers, Manuscripts and Archives Division, New York Public Library, Astor, Lenox, and Tilden Foundations.

Eichhorn, Kate. *The Archival Turn in Feminism: Outrage in Order*. Philadelphia: Temple UP, 2013.

Elman, Julie Passanante. "Cripping Safe Sex: *Life Goes On*'s Queer/Disabled Alliances." *Bioethical Inquiry* 9 (2012): 317–26.

Eng, David. *The Feeling of Kinship: Queer Liberalisim and the Racialization of Intimacy*. Durham: Duke UP, 2010.

Episalla, Joy. Interview by Sarah Schulman. *ACT UP Oral History Project*. Interview no. 036. 6 Dec. 2003. http://actuporalhistory.org/interviews/images/episalla.pdf. Accessed 13 May 2009.Epstein, Julia. "AIDS, Stigma, and Narratives of Containment." *American Imago* 49.3 (Fall 1992): 293–310.

———. *Altered Conditions: Disease, Medicine, and Storytelling*. New York: Routledge, 1995.

Epstein, Steven. *Impure Science: AIDS, Activism, and the Politics of Knowledge*. Berkeley: U of California P, 1996.

Erevelles, Nirmala. "Crippin' Jim Crow: Disability, Dis-Location, and the School-to-Prison Pipeline." In *Disability Incarcerated: Imprisonment and Disability in the United States and Canada*, ed. Liat Ben-Moshe, Chris Chapman, and Allison C. Carey. New York: Palgrave Macmillan, 2014. 81–100.

Erickson, Loree. Interview. Youtube, 2015. https://www.youtube.com/watch?v=SpFvCvFO-jI. Accessed 12 Jan. 2018.

———. "Out of Line: The Sexy Femmegimp Politics of Flaunting It!" In *The Feminist Porn Book: The Politics of Producing Pleasure*, ed. Tristan Taormino, Constance Penley, Celine Parrenas Shimizu, and Mireille Miller-Young. New York: Feminist Press at CUNY, 2013. 320–28.

———. "Revealing Femmegimp: A Sex-Positive Reflection on Sites of Shame as Sites of Resistance for People with Disabilities." *Atlantis* 31.2 (2007): 42–52.

———, dir., actor. *Want*. 2006.

Eswaran, Nisha [nisha.be]. "It's not surprising but I'm so fucking grumpy about the academic response . . ." *Instagram*. 20 Apr. 2020. https://www.instagram.com/p/B

_NQdV8AyapqWb-xDJKH1DimAo3azx3vgblQXwo/?igshid=1cecvmtf2y9h8. Accessed 23 Apr. 2020.

Falconer, Dionne A. Interview by Alexis Shotwell and Gary Kinsman. *AIDS Activist History Project* 1 Apr. 2016. https://aidsactivisthistory.files.wordpress.com/2016/11/aahp -dionne-falconer.pdf. Accessed 16 Apr. 2018.

Farber, Celia. *Serious Adverse Effects: An Uncensored History of AIDS*. Hoboken, NJ: Melville, 2006.

Farmer, Paul. *Infections and Inequalities: The Modern Plagues*. Berkeley: U of California P, 1999.

———. Introduction. In *Global AIDS: Myths and Facts: Tools for Fighting the AIDS Pandemic*, ed. Alexander Irwin, Joyce Millen, and Dorothy Fallows. Cambridge: South End, 2003. xvii–xxiv.

Farrell, Jeanette. *Invisible Enemies: Stories of Infectious Disease*. New York: Farrar, 1998.

Farrow, Kenyon. "When My Brother Fell, Again." *We Who Feel Differently Journal*, ed. Tedd Kerr, 3 (Fall 2014). http://wewhofeeldifferently.info/journal.php.

Fawaz, Ramzi. "I Cherish My Bile Duct as Much as Any Other Organ: Political Disgust and the Digestive Life of AIDS in Tony Kushner's *Angels in America*." *GLQ: A Journal of Lesbian and Gay Studies* 21.1 (2015): 121–52.

Fee, Elizabeth, and Daniel M. Fox. "Introduction: The Contemporary Historiography of AIDS." In *AIDS: The Making of a Chronic Disease*, by Fee and Fox. Berkeley: U of California P, 1992. 1–22.

Feinberg, David. *Queer and Loathing: Rants and Raves of a Raging AIDS Clone*. New York: Penguin, 1994.

Feinberg, Leslie. *Stone Butch Blues*. Ithaca, NY: Firebrand Books, 1993.

Finkelstein, Avram. "AIDS 2.0" *Artwrit*, Dec. 2012. http://www.artwrit.com/article/aids -2-0/. Accessed 2 Feb. 2014.

———. "Silence=_____". *FUSE Magazine*, in conversation with Alex McClelland and Geneviève Trudel, Sept. 2013. fusemagazine.org/2013/09/silenceequals. Accessed 5 Feb. 2014.

Foege, William H. "The Changing Priorities of the Center for Disease Control." *Public Health Reports (1974–), Association of Schools of Public Health* 93.6 (Nov.–Dec. 1978): 616–21.

Ford, Olivia. "*This Positive Life*: Cecilia Chung on Violence, Gender, Prisons, Family and Healing." *The Body* 16 May 2013. www.thebody.com/content/71526/this-positive-life -cecilia-chung-on-violence-gende.html. Accessed 23 June 2018.

Foster, Vanessa Edwards. "President's Ponderings." *Gulf Coast Transgender Community: An Outreach Organization* 11.5 (May 1998): 1. Transgender Archives, University of Victoria. Victoria, British Columbia, Canada.

Foucault, Michel. *The History of Sexuality*. Vol. 1, trans. Robert Hurley. New York: Vintage, 1978.

Freiwald, Bina Toledo. "Becoming and Be/longing: Kate Bornstein's *Gender Outlaw* and *My Gender Workbook*." *Biography* 24.1 (Winter 2001): 35–56.

Fullwood, Steven G. "Our Stories, Our Responsibility." *Metanoia: Transformation through AIDS Archives and Activism*. New York: Self-published exhibit guide, 2019.

Garland-Thomson, Rosemarie. *Staring: How We Look*. Oxford: Oxford UP, 2009.

Garnet Jones, Adam, dir. *Secret Weapons*. CFMDC, 2008. www.cfmdc.org/film/3252.

Garvey, Johanna X. K. "Complicating Categories: 'Race' and Sexuality in Caribbean Women's Fiction." *Journal of Commonwealth and Postcolonial Studies* 10.1 (2003): 94–119.

"GCTC Transmission Line." *Gulf Coast Transgender Community: An Outreach Organization* 8.3 (Mar. 1995): 5–6. Transgender Archives, University of Victoria. Victoria, British Columbia, Canada.

———. *Gulf Coast Transgender Community: An Outreach Organization.* Jan. 1991. Transgender Archives, University of Victoria. Victoria, British Columbia, Canada.

———. *Gulf Coast Transgender Community: An Outreach Organization.* July 1993. Transgender Archives, University of Victoria. Victoria, British Columbia, Canada.

Geary, Adam M. *Antiblack Racism and the AIDS Epidemic: State Intimacies.* New York: Palgrave Macmillan, 2014.

Gillett, James. *A Grassroots History of the HIV/AIDS Epidemic in North America.* Spokane, WA: Marquette, 2011.

Gill-Peterson, Jules. "Haunting the Queer Spaces of AIDS: Remembering ACT UP/New York and an Ethics for an Endemic." *GLQ: A Journal of Lesbian and Gay Studies* 19.3 (2013): 279–300.

———. *Histories of the Transgender Child.* Minneapolis: U of Minnesota P, 2018.

Gilman, Sander L. "AIDS and Syphilis: The Iconography of Disease." In *AIDS: Cultural Analysis Cultural Activism*, ed. Douglas Crimp. Cambridge: MIT P, 1988. 87–108.

Glave, Thomas. "Introduction: Desire through the Archipelago." In *Our Caribbean: A Gathering of Lesbian and Gay Writing from the Antilles* by Glave. Durham: Duke UP, 2008. 1–12.

Goddu, Teresa A. *Gothic America: Narrative, History, and Nation.* New York: Columbia UP, 1997.

Gomez, Jewelle. "Recasting the Mythology: Writing Vampire Fiction." In *Blood Read: The Vampire as Metaphor in Contemporary Culture*, ed. Joan Gordon and Veronica Hollinger. Philadelphia: U of Pennsylvania P, 1997. 85–93.

Gordon, Joan, and Veronica Hollinger. "Introduction: The Shape of Vampires." In *Blood Read: The Vampire as Metaphor in Contemporary Culture*, ed. Joan Gordon and Veronica Hollinger. Philadelphia: U of Pennsylvania P, 1997. 1–10.

Gorna, Robin. *Vamps, Virgins, and Victims: How Can Women Fight AIDS?* London: Cassel, 1996.

Goss, John, dir. *Stiff Sheets.* 1989.

Gossett, Che, and Alice O'Malley. *Duets: Che Gossett & Alice O'Malley in Conversation on Chloe Dzubilo.* Visual AIDS, 2014.

Gould, Deborah B. *Moving Politics: Emotion and ACT UP's Fight against AIDS.* Chicago: U of Chicago P, 2009.

Gran Fury. *AIDS: The Artists' Response.* Ohio State University, 1989. 4.1. Gran Fury Collection, Manuscripts and Archives Division, New York Public Library, Astor, Lenox, and Tilden Foundations.

Gremk, Mirko D. *History of AIDS.* Trans. Russell C. Maulitz and Jacalyn Duffin. Princeton: Princeton UP, 1990.

Greyson, John, dir. *The ADS Epidemic.* 1987.

Grover, Jan Zita. "AIDS: Keywords." In *AIDS: Cultural Analysis Cultural Activism*, ed. Douglas Crimp. Cambridge: MIT P, 1988. 17–30.

Guess, Carol. "Rebecca Brown." Review of *The Gifts of the Body*, by Rebecca Brown. *Lambda Book Report* 15.3 (Fall 2007): 6–7.

Gund, Catherine. Interview by Sarah Schulman. *ACT UP Oral History Project*. Interview no. 071. 20 Apr. 2007. http://actuporalhistory.org/interviews/images/gund.pdf. Accessed 8 Sept. 2011.

Gund, Catherine, and Debra Levine, dirs. *I'm You, You're Me*. Aubin Pictures, 1993.

———. *The Katrina Haslip Memorial Tape*. 1992. AIDS Activist Videotape Collection, Manuscripts and Archives Division, New York Public Library, Astor, Lenox, and Tilden Foundations.

Halberstam, Jack. *In a Queer Time and Place: Transgender Bodies, Subcultural Lives*. New York: NYU P, 2005.

Hallas, Roger. *Reframing Bodies: AIDS, Bearing Witness, and the Queer Moving Image*. Durham: Duke UP, 2009.

Hamel, Kris. "Campaign to Free CeCe McDonald Continues." *Workers World*, 2012. www.workers.org/2012/us/cece_mcdonald_0524/. Accessed 31 May 2012.

Hanhardt, Christina B. *Safe Space: Gay Neighborhood History and the Politics of Violence*. Durham: Duke UP, 2013.

Hanson, Ellis. "Undead." In *Inside/Out: Lesbian Theories, Gay Theories*, ed. Diana Fuss. New York: Routledge, 1991. 324–40.

Hartman, Saidiya. *Wayward Lives, Beautiful Experiments: Intimate Histories of Social Upheaval*. New York: Norton, 2019.

Hastings, Colin. (Panel speaker). "We Can't Police Our Way Out of the Pandemic." Zoom Meeting, 28 Mar. 2020. https://youtu.be/j6s_FZu9F1s?t=5363. Accessed 25 Apr. 2020.

Hebert, Pato. "Forward". *Corpus*, ed. Jamie Cortez and Pato Hebert, 5.1 (Fall 2007): v–xi.

Hernandez, Jasmin. "In Conversation with Kia LaBeija: Using Positivity to Trigger Awareness, Acceptance and Activism for HIV/AIDS." *Gallery Gurls*, 21 Dec. 2015. gallerygurls.net/interviews/2015/12/21/in-conversation-with-kia-labeija-using-positivity-to-trigger-awareness-acceptance-and-activism-for-hivaids. Accessed 11 May 2018.

Herndl, Diane Price. "The Invisible (Invalid) Woman: African-American Women, Illness, and Nineteenth-Century Narrative." *Women's Studies* 24 (1995): 553–72.

Hewitt, Warren W., Jr. "The Healer, Dr. Beny Primm: Uncommon Man for Uncommon Times." In *HIV Pioneers: Lives Lost Careers Changed and Survival*," ed. Wendee M. Wechsberg. Baltimore: RTI, 2018. 16–23.

Hilderbrand, Lucas. "Retroactivism." *GLQ: A Journal of Lesbian and Gay Studies* 12.2 (2006): 303–17.

Hobart, Hi'ilei Julia Kawehipuaakahaopulani, and Tamara Kneese. "Radical Care: Survival Strategies for Uncertain Times." *Social Text* 38.1.142 (Mar. 2020): 1–16.

Hobson, Emily. *Lavender and Red: Liberation and Solidarity in the Gay and Lesbian Left*. Oakland: U of California P, 2016.

———. "Thinking Transnationally, Thinking Queer." In *The Routledge History of Queer America*, ed. Don Romesburg. New York: Routledge, 2018. 200–206.

Hoffman, Amy. *Hospital Time*. Durham: Duke UP, 1997.

Hogan, Katie. *Women Take Care: Gender, Race, and the Culture of AIDS*. Ithaca: Cornell UP, 2001.

Holland, Sharon P. *The Erotic Life of Racism*. Durham: Duke UP, 2012.

Hollibaugh, Amber, Mitchell Karp, and Katy Taylor. "The Second Epidemic." *AIDS: Cultural Analysis/Cultural Activism*, special issue of *October* 43 (Winter, 1987): 127–42.

Holmes, Trevor. "Coming Out of the Coffin: Gay Males and Queer Goths in Contemporary Vampire Fiction." In *Blood Read: The Vampire as Metaphor in Contemporary Culture*, ed. Joan Gordon and Veronica Hollinger. Philadelphia: U of Pennsylvania P, 1997. 169–88.

Hoolbloom, Mike, dir. *Frank's Cock*. (Independent Production), 1993.

Hoppe, Trevor. *Punishing Disease: HIV and the Criminalization of Sickness*. Oakland: U of California P, 2018.

Hwang, Ren-Yo. "Deviant Care for Deviant Futures: QTBIPoC Radical Realtionism as Mutual Aid against Carceral Care." *Transgender Studies Quarterly* 6.4 (Nov. 2019): 559–78.

"In the News." *En Femme Magazine* 8 (Sept.–Oct. 1988): 38–39. Transgender Archives, University of Victoria. Victoria, British Columbia, Canada.

"Internet Archive." *Outweek*. outweek.net. Accessed 30 May 2012.

Israel, Gianna E. "Post-Op Living." *Trans-Port: A Peer Support Group for All Transgendered Individuals* (July 1997). Transgender Archives, University of Victoria. Victoria, British Columbia, Canada.

Jackson, Emma, Chanelle Gallant, Annie Morgan Banks, Johanna Lewis, and Sheryle Carlson. "Five Ways to Take Anti-Racist Action During COVID-19." *TheTyee.ca*. 10 Apr. 2020. https://thetyee.ca/Opinion/2020/04/10/Five-Ways-To-Take-Anti-Racist-Action-During -COVID-19/. Accessed 24 Apr. 2020.

Jaspal, Rusi, Lauren Kennedy, and Shema Tariq. "Human Immunodeficiency Virus and Trans Women: A Literature Review." *Transgender Health* 3.1 (2019): 239–50.

Jiwani, Yasmin, and Mary Lynn Young. "Missing and Murdered Women: Reproducing Marginality in News Discourse." *Canadian Journal of Communication* 31 (2006): 895–917.

Johnson, E. Patrick. "'Quare' Studies, Or (Almost) Everything I Know about Queer Studies I Learned from My Grandmother." In *Black Queer Studies: A Critical Anthology*, ed. E. Patrick Johnson and Mae G. Henderson. Durham: Duke UP, 2005. 124–59.

Jones, El. (Panel speaker). "We Can't Police Our Way Out of the Pandemic." Zoom Meeting, 28 Mar. 2020. https://youtu.be/j6s_FZu9F1s?t=1583. Accessed 25 Apr. 2020.

Jones, James H. *Bad Blood: The Tuskegee Syphilis Experiment*. New York: Free Press, 1981.

Jones, James W. "Refusing the Name: The Absence of AIDS in Recent American Gay Male Fiction." In *Writing AIDS: Gay Literature, Language, and Analysis*, ed. Timothy F. Murphy and Suzanne Poirier. New York: Columbia UP, 1993. 225–43.

Jones, Miriam. "*The Gilda Stories*: Revealing the Monsters at the Margins." In *Blood Read: The Vampire as Metaphor in Contemporary Culture*, ed. Joan Gordon and Veronica Hollinger. Philadelphia: U of Pennsylvania P, 1997. 151–67.

Jordan, Taryn. *The Politics of Impossibility: CeCe McDonald and Trayvon Martin—the Bursting of Black Rage*. MA thesis. Georgia State University, 2014. *ScholarWorks*. scholarworks.gsu.edu/cgi/viewcontent.cgi?article=1046&context=wsi_theses. Accessed 15 May 2016.

Jordan-Zachery, Julia S. "Safe, Soulful Sex: HIV/AIDS Talk." In *AIDS and the Distribution of Crises*, ed. Jih-Fei Cheng, Alexandra Juhasz, and Nishant Shahani. Durham: Duke UP, 2020. 93–130.

Joynt, Chase and Mike Hoolbloom. *You Only Live Twice: Sex, Death, and Transition*. Toronto: Coach House, 2016.

Juhasz, Alexandra. *AIDS TV: Identity, Community, and Alternative Video*. Durham: Duke UP, 1995.

———. "The Contained Threat: Women in Mainstream AIDS Documentary." *Journal of Sex Research* 27.1 (Feb. 1990): 25–46.

———. "Feminist History Making and Video Remains." *Jump Cut*, in exchange with Antoinette Burton, 48 (Winter 2006). http://www.ejumpcut.org/archive/jc48.2006/AIDsJuhasz/.

———. "Introduction." *What Does a COVID-19 Doula Do?* (Online Zine). One Archives, Mar. 2020. https://www.onearchives.org/what-does-a-covid19-doula-do-zine/. Accessed 25 Apr. 2020.

———. "Video Remains: Nostalgia, Technology, and Queer Archive Activism." *GLQ: A Journal of Lesbian and Gay Studies* 12.2 (2006): 319–28.

———. "When ACT UP Is Remembered . . . Other Places, People, and Forms of AIDS Activism Are Disremembered." Blog entry. *Visual AIDS*. 17 Feb. 2013. visualaids.org/blog/detail/7414. Accessed 9 Nov. 2013.

Juhasz, Alexandra, Jih-Fei Cheng, Lucas Hilderbrand, Adam Geary, Theodore Kerr, Nishant Shahani, and Dagmawi Woubshet. "A Political Sense of Being at Home with HIV and Video." *AIDS and Memory*, special issue of *Drain*, with Amber Dean, ed. Ricky Varghese, 14.2 (2016). drainmag.com/a-political-sense-of-being-at-home-with-hiv-and-video/. Accessed 10 July 2017.

Juhasz, Alexandra, and Ted Kerr. "Home Video Returns: Media Ecologies of the Past of HIV/AIDS." *Cineaste* 39.3 (2014). https://www.cineaste.com/summer2014/home-video-returns-media-ecologies-of-the-past-of-hiv-aids.

Jung, Katie. *Forget Burial*. Silkscreen art collaboration with Marty Fink. Concordia University, 2013.

Kafer, Alison. *Feminist, Queer, Crip*. Bloomington: U of Indiana P, 2013.

Keeler, Doug. "Sharps Container Ghosts." *Helix Queer Performance Network*. 30 Oct. 2014. helixqpn.org/post/101379965247/sharps-container-ghosts. Accessed 29 May 2018.

Kelly, Bryn. "The HIV Welfare Merry-Go-Round: A Day in the Life." Blog entry. *Partybottom: The *Sexy* HIV+ Transgender Blog*. 1 Aug. 2014. *Tumblr*. partybottom.tumblr.com/post/93524746788/the-hiv-welfare-merry-go-round-a-day-in-the-life. Accessed 8 Nov. 2017.

———. "How to Be a Good Roommate to Someone Living with HIV/AIDS." Blog entry. *Partybottom: The *Sexy* HIV+ Transgender Blog*. 12 Jan. 2014. *Tumblr*. partybottom.tumblr.com/post/73161473477/how-to-be-a-good-roommate-to-someone-living-with. Accessed 8 Nov. 2017.

———. "I Went to the Doctor Yesterday . . ." Blog entry. *Partybottom: The *Sexy* HIV+ Transgender Blog*. 30 May 2014. *Tumblr*. partybottom.tumblr.com/post/87329854418/i-went-to-the-doctor-yesterday-started#notes. Accessed 7 Nov. 2017.

———. "Ok, Time to Blow Up Someone's Spot." Blog entry. *Partybottom: The *Sexy* HIV+ Transgender Blog*. 18 Aug. 2014. *Tumblr*. https://partybottom.tumblr.com/post/95140228633/ok-time-to-blow-up-someones-spot. Accessed 7 Nov. 2017.

———. "Other Balms, Other Gileads." *We Who Feel Differently Journal*, ed. Tedd Kerr, 3 (Fall 2014). http://wewhofeeldifferently.info/journal.php#Bryn.

———. "Partybottom: The *Sexy* HIV+ Transgender Blog." *Tumblr*. Dec. 2013–Nov. 2015. partybottom.tumblr.com/. Accessed 7 Nov. 2017.

————. "Prep Might Not Be the Aanswer but, Hey, It's Worth a Shot." *Bryn Kelly*. 3 Dec. 2013. *Tumblr*. brynkelly.tumblr.com/post/68807862615/prep-might-not-be-the-answer-but-hey-its-worth. Accessed 8 Nov. 2017.

————. "A Tale of Two Trans Care Program Case Managers." Blog entry. *Partybottom: The *Sexy* HIV+ Transgender Blog*. 13 Dec. 2013. *Tumblr*. partybottom.tumblr.com/post/69912399178/a-tale-of-two-trans-care-program-case-managers#notes. Accessed 8 Nov. 2017.

————. "Your Life Is Worth Living Even If . . ." Blog entry. *Partybottom: The *Sexy* HIV+ Transgender Blog*. 29 May 2014. *Tumblr*. partybottom.tumblr.com/post/87236802443/your-life-is-worth-living-even-if-youre-not#notes. Accessed 7 Nov. 2017.

Kelly, Christine, and Michael Orsini. "Introduction: Mobilizing Metaphor." In *Mobilizing Metaphor: Art, Culture, and Disability Activism in Canada*, by Kelly and Orsini. Vancouver: UBC Press, 2016. 3–21.

Kerr, Ted. "AIDS 1969: HIV, History, and Race." *AIDS and Memory*, special issue of *Drain*, with Amber Dean, ed. Ricky Varghese, 14.2 (2016). drainmag.com/aids-1969-hiv-history-and-race/. Accessed 10 July 2017.

————. "How to Live With a Virus." *POZ*. 23 Mar. 2020. https://www.poz.com/article/live-virus. Accessed on 22 Apr. 2020.

————. (Panel speaker). "We Can't Police Our Way Out of the Pandemic." Zoom Meeting, 28 Mar. 2020. https://youtu.be/j6s_FZu9F1s?t=5954. Accessed 25 Apr. 2020.

————. "Who Is HIV For?" *Women's Studies Quarterly* 42.3/4 (Fall/Winter 2014): 333–38.

Kerr, Theodore (Ted), Catherine Yuk-ping Lo, Ian Bradley-Perrin, Sarah Schlman, and Eric A. Stanley with an Introduction by Nishant Shahani. "Dispatches on the Globalizations of AIDS." In *AIDS and the Distribution of Crises*, ed. Jih-Fei Cheng, Alexandra Juhasz, and Nishant Shahani. Durham: Duke UP, 2020. 29–59

Kilgore, De Witt Douglass. "Beyond the History We Know: Nnedi Okorafor-Mbachu, Nisi Shawl, and Jarla Tangh Rethink Science Fiction Tradition." In *Afro-Future Females: Black Writers Chart Science Fiction's Newest New-Wave Trajectory*, ed. Marleen S. Barr. Columbus: Ohio State UP, 2008. 119–29.

Kimoto, Diane M. "Affirming the Role of Women as Carers: The Social Construction of AIDS through the Eyes of Mother, Friend, and Nurse." In *Women and AIDS: Negotiating Safer Practices, Care, and Representation*, ed. Nancy L. Roth and Linda K. Fuller. Binghamton: Harrington Park, 1998. 155–80.

Kincaid, Jamaica. *My Brother*. New York: Farrar, 1997.

Kinsman, Gary. (Panel speaker). "We Can't Police Our Way Out of the Pandemic." Zoom Meeting, 28 Mar. 2020. https://youtu.be/AK9ioHaTu38?t=2443. Accessed 25 Apr. 2020.

Knauer, Nancy J. "LGBT Older Adults, Chosen Family, and Caregiving." *Journal of Law and Religion* 31.2 (2016): 150–68.

Kohnen, Melanie E. S. *Queer Representation, Visibility, and Race in American Film and Television: Screening the Closet*. New York: Routledge, 2015.

Konsmo, Erin Marie. "'Art through a Birch Bark Heart': An Illustrated Interview with Erin Marie Konsmo (with PJ Lilley)." *Radical Criminology* 2 (2013). journal.radicalcriminology.org/index.php/rc/article/view/29/html. Accessed 4 May 2017.

Köppert, Katrin, and Todd Sekuler. "Sick Memory: On the Un-detectable in Archiving Aids." *AIDS and Memory*, special issue of *Drain*, with Amber Dean, ed. Ricky Varghese, 14.2 (2016). drainmag.com/sick-memory-on-the-un-detectable-in-archiving-aids/. Accessed 10 July 2017.

Kramer, Larry. *Reports from the Holocaust*. New York: St. Martin's, 1997.

Krishtalka, Sholem. "Art-Led Activism Wins the AIDS Day." *Toronto Standard* 17 Mar. 2011. http://www.torontostandard.com/culture/artist-led-activism-wins-the-aids -day/. Accessed 12 Apr. 2011.

Kruger, Steven F. *AIDS Narratives: Gender and Sexuality, Fiction and Science*. New York: Garland, 1996.

LaBeija, Kia. "Ajamu's Curatorial Residency." *Visual AIDS*. 2016. *Vimeo*. vimeo.com /161956845.

———. "Artist's Statement." Blog entry. *Visual AIDS*. 19 Oct. 2015. www.visualaids.org /blog/detail/kia-labeija-eleven. Accessed 10 June 2017.

———. "24." In *Art AIDS America*, ed. Jonathan D. Katz, and Rock Hushka. Seattle, WA: U of Washington P, 2015. 273.

LaBeija, Kia, and Julie Tolentino. *Duets: Kia LaBeija and Julie Tolentino in Conversation*. New York: Visual AIDS, 2018

Lakshmi Piepzna-Samarasinha, Leah. *Care Work: Dreaming Disability Justice*. Vancouver: Arsenal, 2018.

Lawler, Michelle, dir. *Forever's Gonna Start Tonight*. Aggressively Enthusiastic Films, 2009.

Lee, Nathan, curator. "Undetectable." Blog entry. *Visual AIDS*. May 2012. visualaids .blogspot.ca/2012/05/undetectable-public-programming.html. Accessed 17 June 2012.

Lee, Nathan, and Carlos Motta. "There Is Tremendous Ferocity in Being Gentle." *We Who Feel Differently Journal*, ed. Tedd Kerr, 3 (Fall 2014). http://wewhofeeldifferently .info/journal.php.

Leigh, Carol. *Unrepentant Whore: The Collected Works of Scarlot Harlot*. San Francisco: Last Gasp, 2004.

Leonard, Zoe. Interview by Sarah Schulman. *ACT UP Oral History Project*. Interview no. 106. 13 Jan. 2010. http://actuporalhistory.org/interviews/images/leonard.pdf. Accessed 3 Mar. 2017.

Levine, Debra. *Demonstrating ACT UP: The Ethics, Politics, and Performances of Affinity*. Dissertation. New York University, 2012.

Levine, Philippa. *Prostitution, Race, and Politics: Policing Venereal Disease in the British Empire*. New York: Routledge, 2003.

Lind, Betty Ann. "Denver IFGE Address for Virginia Prince Award." *Our Sorority* 26 (Sept. 1991): 5–24. Transgender Archives, University of Victoria. Victoria, British Columbia, Canada.

———. "The Future of The Outreach Institute: On the Order of Being: A Progress Report." *Our Sorority* 21 (Jan. 1990): 3–10. Transgender Archives, University of Victoria. Victoria, British Columbia, Canada.

Linton, Simi. "Reassigning Meaning." In *The Disability Studies Reader*, ed. Lennard J. Davis, 2nd ed. New York: Routledge, 2006, 161–72.

Liss, Sarah. *Army of Lovers: A Community History of Will Munro*. Toronto: Coach House, 2013.

Long, Thomas L. *AIDS and American Apocalypticism: The Cultural Semiotics of an Empire*. Albany, NY: State U of New York P, 2005.

Lorde, Audre. *The Cancer Journals*. San Francisco: Aunt Lute, 1980.

Love, Heather. *Feeling Backward: Loss and the Politics of Queer History*. Cambridge: Harvard UP, 2007.

Loyd, Jenna M., Matt Mitchelson, and Andrew Burridge. "Introduction: Borders, Prisons, and Abolitionist Visions." In *Beyond Walls and Cages: Prisons, Borders, and Global Crisis*, ed. Jenna M. Loyd, Matt Mitchelson, and Andrew Burridge. Athens: U of Georgia P, 2012. 1–18.

Lundberg, Elizabeth. "Let Me Bite You Again: Vampiric Agency in Octavia Butler's *Fledgling*." *GLQ: A Journal of Lesbian and Gay Studies* 21.4 (2015): 561–84.

Ma, Ming Yuen S. "Interview by Sarah Schulman. *ACT UP Oral History Project*. Interview no. 007. 15 Jan. 2003. http://actuporalhistory.org/interviews/images/ma.pdf. Accessed 8 Mar. 2017.

Mackay, Xanthra Phillippa. "Don't Touch Me—I'm Electric TS Epileptic." *Gender Trash from Hell*. Issue 3. Genderpress, 1995.

———. "TRANSSEXUALS / GET / AIDS / TOO . . ." *Gender Trash from Hell*. Issue 1. Genderpress, 1993.

Mackay, Xanthra Phillippa, and Ross, Mirha-Soleil, eds. *Gender Trash from Hell*. Issue 1. Genderpress, 1993.

Mackenzie, Sonja. *Structural Intimacies: Sexual Stories from the Black AIDS Epidemic*. New Brunswick: Rutgers UP, 2013.

Maher, JaneMaree, Sharon Pickering, and Alison Gerard. *Sex Work: Labour, Mobility, and Sexual Services*. New York: Routledge, 2013.

Marcus, Sharon. "Queer Theory for Everyone: A Review Essay." *Signs: Journal of Women in Culture and Society* 31.1 (2005): 191–218.

Marshall, Stuart. "Picturing Deviancy." In *Ecstatic Antibodies: Resisting the AIDS Mythology*, ed. Tessa Boffin and Sunil Gupta. London: Rivers Oram, 1990. 19–36.

Mass, Larry. Interview. *GMHC Oral History Project*. Interview 00944-ABC. AIDS Activist Videotape Collection. Manuscripts and Archives Division, New York Public Library, Astor, Lenox, and Tilden Foundations.

Maynard, Robyn. *Policing Black Lives: State Violence in Canada from Slavery to the Present*. Halifax: Fernwood, 2017.

Maynard, Robyn, and Andrea J. Ritchie. "Black Communities Need Support, Not a Coronavirus Police State." Vice. (Online). 9 Apr. 2020. https://www.vice.com/en_ca/article/z3bdmx/black-people-coronavirus-police-state?. Accessed 24 Apr. 2020.

McCarthy, Margaret, and David Kirschenbaum. "A Mandatory Test by Any Other Name: New Jersey's Attack on Women with HIV." *Outweek* 18 (22 Oct. 1989): 34–35. Lesbian Herstory Archives. Brooklyn, NY.

McCaskell, Tim. *Queer Progress: From Homophobia to Homonationalism*. Toronto: Between the Lines, 2016.

McClelland, Alexander. "Unprepared." *Maisonneuve* 71 (Spring 2019): 40–45.

———. "We Can't Police Our Way Out of a Pandemic." *Now Magazine*. 30 Mar. 2020. https://nowtoronto.com/news/coronavirus-we-cant-police-our-way-out-of-pandemic. Accessed 22 Apr. 2020.

———. (Panel speaker). "We Can't Police Our Way Out of the Pandemic." Zoom Meeting, 28 Mar. 2020. https://youtu.be/j6s_FZu9F1s. Accessed 25 Apr. 2020.

McClelland, Alexander, and Jessica Whitbread. "PosterVirus: Claiming Sexual Autonomy for People with HIV through Collective Action." In *Mobilizing Metaphor: Art, Culture, and Disability Activism in Canada*, ed. Christine Kelly and Michael Orsini. Vancouver: UBC Press, 2016. 76–97.

McGrath, Mark, and Bob Sutcliffe. "Insuring Profits from AIDS: The Economics of an Epidemic." *Facing AIDS: A Special Issue*, special issue of *Radical America*, 20.6 (1987): 9–27. Lesbian Herstory Archives. Brooklyn, NY.

McKenzie, Vivian. "February Meeting." *Gulf Coast Transgender Community: An Outreach Organization* 9.3 (Mar. 1996). Transgender Archives, University of Victoria. Victoria, British Columbia, Canada.

McKinney, Cait. "Can a Computer Remember AIDS?" *AIDS and Memory*, special issue of *Drain*, with Amber Dean, ed. Ricky Varghese, 14.2 (2016). drainmag.com/can-a -computer-remember-aids/. Accessed 10 July 2017.

———. "Printing Out the Internet: AIDS Activism from Online Bulletin Boards to Print Newsletters." *Thinking beyond Backlash: Remediating 1980s Activisms*, 28 May 2017. Women's and Gender Studies et Recherches Féministes, Toronto.

McKinney, Cait, and Hazel Meyer. *Tape Condition: Degraded*. The Canadian Lesbian and Gay Archives and Push Rub Press, 2016.

McRuer, Robert. *Crip Theory: Cultural Signs of Queerness and Disability*. New York: NYU P, 2006.

———. "Critical Investments: AIDS, Christopher Reeve, and Queer/Disability Studies." *Journal of Medical Humanities* 23, nos. 3–4 (2002): 226.

———. "Disability and the NAMES Project." *Public Historian* 27.2 (Spring 2005): 53–61.

Mehaffy, Marilyn, and AnaLouise Keating. "'Radio Imagination': Octavia Butler on the Poetics of Narrative Embodiment." *Melus* 26.1 (Spring 2001): 45–77.

The Members of the ACE Program (AIDS Counseling and Education) of the Bedford Hills Correctional Facility. *Breaking the Walls of Silence: AIDS and Women in a New York State Maximum-Security Prison*. Woodstock, NY: Overlook, 1998.

Metzl, Jonathan. "Introduction: Why 'Against Health'?" In *Against Health: How Health Became the New Morality*, ed. Jonathan Metzl and Anna Kirkland. New York: NYU P, 2010. 1–13.

Mikiki, Mikiki. "I Party/ I Bareback/ I'm Positive/ I'm Responsible." *PosterVirus*, with Scott Donald, AAN Toronto, 2011.

———. Interview by Nicholas Little. "The Party of Not Talking about It—Nicholas Little with Mikiki." *No More Potlucks*, No. 8: Beast, Mar.–Apr. 2010. nomorepotlucks.org/site /the-party-of-not-talking-about-it. Accessed 19 Nov. 2011.

———, Perf. *These Conversations but with People We're Hot For*. Video documentation from *Down in a Blaze of Glory Hole*, 2007.

———. (Panel speaker). "We Can't Police Our Way Out of the Pandemic." Zoom Meeting, 28 Mar. 2020. https://youtu.be/j6s_FZu9F1s?t=2382. Accessed 25 Apr. 2020.

Miller, Nancy K. *But Enough about Me: Why We Read Other People's Lives*. New York: Columbia UP, 2002.

Miner, Valerie. Review of *The Gifts of the Body* by Rebecca Brown and *Who Will Run the Frog Hospital?* by Lorrie Moore Source. *Women's Review of Books* 12.7 (Apr. 1995): 14–15.

Mingus, Mia. "Access Intimacy, Interdependence and Disability Justice." Paul K. Longmore Lecture on Disability Studies, 11 Apr. 2017, San Francisco. *WordPress*. https:// leavingevidence.wordpress.com/2017/04/12/access-intimacy-interdependence-and -disability-justice/. Accessed 6 May 2019.

———. "Moving toward the Ugly: A Politic beyond Desirability." Femmes of Color Symposium, 21 Aug. 2011, Oakland. Keynote address. *WordPress*. leavingevidence

.wordpress.com/2011/08/22/moving-toward-the-ugly-a-politic-beyond-desirability/. Accessed 4 May 2019.

"Mirha-Soleil Ross (1969–) Sex Worker, Activist, Performer, Filmmaker, Broadcaster." Blog entry. *A Gender Variance Who's Who*. 24 Sept. 2014. zagria.blogspot.ca/2014/09 /mirha-soleil-ross-1969-sex-worker.html#.WZSu9tPytE4. Accessed 23 Mar. 2018.

Mirza, Mansha. "Refugee Camps, Asylum Detention, and the Geopolitics of Transnational Migration: Disability and Its Intersections with Humanitarian Confinement." In *Disability Incarcerated: Imprisonment and Disability in the United States and Canada*, ed. Liat Ben-Moshe, Chris Chapman, and Allison C. Carey. New York: Palgrave Macmillan, 2014. 217–36.

"Mission Statement." *City Lights*, 18 Nov. 2008. www.citylights.com/publishing/?fa =publishing_mission. Accessed 20 June 2009.

Mitchell, Allyson, and Jessica Whitbread. "Fuck Positive Women." *PosterVirus*, AAN Toronto, 2011.

Mitchell, Ned. "Sexual, Ethnic, National, and Disabled Identities in the 'Borderlands' of Latino/a America and African America." In *Blackness and Disability: Critical Examinations and Cultural Interventions*, ed. Chris Bell. East Lansing: Michigan State UP, 2012. 113–26.

Mock, Janet. *Redefining Realness: My Path to Womanhood, Identity, Love, and So Much More*. New York: Atria, 2014.

Mogul, Joey L., Andrea J. Ritchie, and Kay Whitlock. *Queer (In)Justice: The Criminalization of LGBT People in the United States*. Boston: Beacon, 2011.

Mollow, Anna. "'When Black Women Start Going on Prozac': The Politics of Race, Gender, and Emotional Distress in Meri Nana-Ama Danquah's *Willow Weep for Me*." *MELUS* 31.3 (2006): 67–99.

Morgensen, Scott Lauria. *Spaces between Us: Queer Settler Colonialism and Indigenous Decolonization*. Minneapolis: U of Minnesota P, 2011.

Morris, David B. "The Plot of Suffering: AIDS and Evil." In *Evil after Postmodernism: Histories, Narratives, and Ethics*, ed. Jennifer L. Geddes. Abingdon, UK: Routledge, 2001. 56–78.

Morris, Susana M. "Black Girls Are from the Future: Afrofuturist Feminism in Octavia E. Butler's *Fledgling*." *Women's Studies Quarterly* 40.3/4 (Fall/Winter 2012): 146–66.

Muñoz, José Esteban. *Cruising Utopia: The Then and There of Queer Futurity*. New York: NYU P, 2009.

———. *Disidentifications: Queers of Color and the Performance of Politics*. Minneapolis: U of Minnesota P, 1999.

Munro, Lauren, Zack Marshall, Greta Bauer, Rebecca Hammond, Caleb Nault, and Robb Travers. "(Dis)integrated Care: Barriers to Health Care Utilization for Trans Women Living with HIV." *Journal of the Association of Nurses in AIDS Care* 28.5 (Sept./ Oct. 2017): 708–22.

Murray, Joseph J, and H-Dirksen L Bauman. "Deaf Gain: An Introduction." In *Deaf Gain: Raising the Stakes for Human Diversity*, ed. H-Dirksen L Bauman and Joseph J Murray. Minneapolis: U of Minnesota P, 2014. xv–xlii.

Mutual Aid Disaster Relief. "Collective Care is our Best Weapon" Online resource guide. Mar. 2020. https://mutualaiddisasterrelief.org/collective-care/. Accessed 24 Apr. 2020.

My Body / My Story: Body Mapping and HIV Treatment Side Effects Project Report. International Community of Women Living with HIV, Apr. 2017.

Namaste, Viviane. "AIDS Histories Otherwise: The Case of Haitians in Montreal." In *AIDS and the Distribution of Crises*, ed. Jih-Fei Cheng, Alexandra Juhasz, and Nishant Shahani. Durham: Duke UP, 2020, 131–47.

———. *Sex Change, Social Change: Reflections on Identity, Institutions, and Imperialism.* Toronto: Women's Press, 2005.

Namaste, Viviane, T H Vukov, Nada Saghie, Robin Williamson, Jacky Vallée, M Lafrenière, M Leroux, Andréa Monette, and Joseph Jean-Gilles. *HIV Prevention and Bisexual Realities.* Toronto: U of Toronto P, 2015.

Nguyen, Vinh-Kim. *The Republic of Therapy: Triage and Sovereignty in West Africa's Time of AIDS.* Durham: Duke UP, 2010.

Nikolas, Akash. "Straight Growth and the Imperial Alternative: Queer-Reading Jamaica Kincaid." *African American Review* 50.1 (Spring 2017): 59–73.

Nixon, Lindsay. "States of Emergency: Confronting the Erasure of Indigenous Women and Two-Spirited People in HIV Movements." *Briarpatch Magazine* 1 Jan. 2017. briarpatchmagazine.com/articles/view/states-of-emergency. Accessed 27 Apr. 2017.

Nixon, Nicola. "When Hollywood Sucks, or, Hungry Girls, Lost Boys, and Vampirism in the Age of Reagan." In *Blood Read: The Vampire as Metaphor in Contemporary Culture*, ed. Joan Gordon and Veronica Hollinger. Philadelphia: U of Pennsylvania P, 1997. 115–28.

Northrop, Ann. Interview by Sarah Schulman. *ACT UP Oral History Project.* Interview no. 027. 28 May 2003. http://actuporalhistory.org/interviews/images/ma.pdf. Accessed 10 Oct. 2008.

Nunokawa, Jeff. "'All the Sad Young Men': AIDS and the Work of Mourning." In *Inside/Out: Lesbian Theories, Gay Theories*, ed. Diana Fuss. New York: Routledge, 1991. 311–23.

Nyong'o, Tavia. *Afro-Fabulations: The Queer Drama of Black Life.* New York: NYU P, 2019.

Oliver, Vanessa, Sarah Flicker, Jessica Danforth, Erin Konsmo, Ciann Wilson, Randy Jackson, Jean-Paul Restoule, Tracey Prentice, June Larkin, and Claudia Mitchell. "'Women Are Supposed To Be the Leaders': Intersections of Gender, Race and Colonisation in HIV Prevention with Indigenous Young People." *Culture, Health & Sexuality* 17.7 (2015): 906–19.

Pacifico de Carvalho, Nathália, Cássia Cristina Pinto Mendicino, Raissa Carolina Fonseca Cândido, Denyr Jeferson Dutra Alecrim, and Cristiane Aparecida Menezes de Pádua. "HIV Pre-exposure Prophylaxis (PrEP) Awareness and Acceptability among Trans Women: A Review." *AIDS Care: Psychological and Socio-medical Aspects of AIDS/HIV* (May 2019): 1–7.

Padilla, Mark. *Caribbean Pleasure Industry: Tourism, Sexuality, and AIDS in the Dominican Republic.* Chicago: U of Chicago P, 2007.

Page, Kezia. "'What If He Did Not Have a Sister [Who Lived in the United States]?' Jamaica Kincaid's *My Brother* as Remittance Text." *small axe* 21 (Oct. 2006): 37–53.

Page, Morgan M. *Brazen: Trans Women's Safer Sex Guide.* Toronto: 519 Church Street Community Centre, 2012.

———. "Odofemi: Sept 26, 2012." *Tumblr.* Sept. 2012. odofemi.tumblr.com/day/2012/09/26. Accessed 8 Jan. 2014.

Page, Morgan M., Jessica Whitbread, Johnny Forever, and Tania Anderson, dirs. "I Don't Need a Spacesuit to Fuck You." 2013. *Vimeo.* vimeo.com/85746077.

Parreñas, Juno Salazar. *Decolonizing Extinction: The Work of Care in Orangutan Rehabilitation*. Durham: Duke UP, 2018.

PASAN/The Canadian AIDS Legal Network. *Hard Time: Promoting HIV and Hepatitis C Prevention Programming for Prisoners in Canada*. Toronto: Canadian AIDS Legal Network, 2007.

Patterson, Kathy Davis. "Haunting Back: Vampire Subjectivity in 'The Gilda Stories.'" *Femspec* 6.1 (2005): 35–57.

Patton, Cindy. "Forward." In *AIDS and the Distribution of Crises*, ed. Jih-Fei Cheng, Alexandra Juhasz, and Nishant Shahani. Durham: Duke UP, 2020, vii–xvi.

———. *Globalizing AIDS*. Minneapolis: U of Minnesota P, 2002.

———. "Resistance and the Erotic: Reclaiming History, Setting Strategy as We Face AIDS." *Facing AIDS: A Special Issue*, special issue of *Radical America*, 20.6 (1987): 68–74. Lesbian Herstory Archives. Brooklyn, NY.

———. "Safe Sex and the Pornographic Vernacular." In *How Do I Look?: Queer Film and Video*, ed. The Bad Object-Choices Collective. Seattle: Bay Press, 1991. 31–63.

Pearl, Monica B. *AIDS Literature and Gay Identity: The Literature of Loss*. New York: Routledge, 2013.

———. "American Grief: The AIDS Quilt and Texts of Witness." *GRAMMA* 16 (2009): 251–72.

Penzenstadler, Kathy, and Alix Birkley. "Fluid Frontiers: AIDS, Vampires, and a Cultural Analysis of Our Fear of Wetness." *Thresholds, Viewing Culture* 7 (1993): 145–48.

Pitts, Victoria. "Visibly Queer: Body Technologies and Sexual Politics." *The Sociological Quarterly* 41.3 (Summer, 2000): 443–63.

Plett, Casey. *A Safe Girl to Love*. New York: Topside, 2014.

Poteat, Tonia C., JoAnne Keatly, Rose Wilcher, and Chloe Schwenke. "Evidence for Action: A Call for the Global HIV Response to Address the Needs of Transgender Populations." *Journal of the International AIDS Society* 19, suppl. 2 (2016): 1–4.

Powder Puffs of California. "Fashion Show/Luncheon." *Girl Talk* 11.4 (Apr. 1996): 1. Transgender Archives, University of Victoria. Victoria, British Columbia, Canada.

———. "From the Internet." *Girl Talk* 11.6 (June 1996): 2. Transgender Archives, University of Victoria. Victoria, British Columbia, Canada.

Powell, Patricia. *A Small Gathering of Bones*. Portsmouth, NH: Heinemann, 1994.

Pros and Cons: A Guide to Creating Successful HIV and HCV Programs for Prisoners. 2nd ed. Toronto: PASAN, 2011.

Puar, Jasbir K. "In the Wake of *It Gets Better*: The Campaign Prompted by Recent Gay Youth Suicides Promotes a Narrow Version of Gay Identity that Risks Further Marginalization." *The Guardian* 16 Nov. 2010. www.guardian.co.uk/commentisfree/cifamerica /2010/nov/16/wake-it-gets-better-campaign. Accessed 22 Jan. 2013.

———. *The Right to Maim: Debility, Capacity, Disability*. Durham: Duke UP, 2017.

———. *Terrorist Assemblages: Homonationalism in Queer Times*. Durham: Duke UP, 2007.

PWA Coalition. "Statement of Prisoners in the AIDS Ward on Rikers Island." In *AIDS: Cultural Analysis Cultural Activism*, ed. Douglas Crimp. Cambridge: MIT P, 1988.

Race, Kane. "Reluctant Objects: Sexual Pleasure as a Problem for HIV Biomedical Prevention." *GLQ: A Journal of Lesbian and Gay Studies* 21.1 (2015): 1–31.

Rahim, Jennifer. "The Operations of the Closet and the Discourse of Unspeakable Contents in *Black Fauns* and *My Brother*." *SX20*, June 2006, 1–18.

Ramirez-Valles, Jesus. *Compañeros: Latino Activists in the Face of AIDS*. Chicago: U of Chicago P, 2011.

Rees, Geoffrey. "The Clinic and the Tea Room." *Journal of Medical Humanities* 34 (2013): 109–21.

Reid-Pharr, Robert. Forward. *Corpus*, by Reid-Pharr, 3.1 (Fall 2005): v–vi.

Rice, Anne P. "Burning Connections: Maternal Betrayal in Jamaica Kincaid's *My Brother*." *A/B: Auto/Biography Studies* 14.1 (1999): 23–37.

Rifkin, Mark. *The Erotics of Sovereignty: Queer Native Writing in the Era of Self-Determination*. Minneapolis: U Minnesota Press, 2012.

Ritchie, Beth. *Arrested Justice: Black Women, Violence, and America's Prison Nation*. New York: NYU P, 2012.

———. "Queering Antiprison Work: African American Lesbians in the Juvenile Justice System." In *Global Lockdown: Race, Gender, and the Prison Industrial Complex*, ed. Julia Sudbury. New York: Routledge, 2005.

Rivera, Sylvia. "Queens in Exile: The Forgotten Ones." In *GenderQueer: Voices from Beyond the Sexual Binary*, ed. Joan Nestle, Clare Howell, and Riki Wilchins. Los Angeles: Alyson, 2002. 67–85.

Robinson, Colin. "An Archaeology of Grief: The Fear of Remembering Joe Beam." In *Black Gay Genius: Answering Joseph Beam's Call*, ed. Steven G. Fullwood and Charles Stephens. New York: Vintage Entity, 2014.

———. "Homophobia Causes AIDS! Pass It On." *The Scarlet Letters* 3.1 (Spring 2006): 7–11.

Rodney, Sur (Sur). "Oral History Interview with Sur Rodney (Sur)." Interview by Ted Kerr. 12 and 15 July 2016. Smithsonian Archives of American Art. https://www.aaa .si.edu/collections/interviews/oral-history-interview-sur-rodney-sur-17369. Accessed 13 July 2018.

Rodriguez, Juana Maria. *Queer Latinidad: Identity Practices, Discursive Spaces*. New York: NYU P, 2003.

Rollerena. Interview by Sarah Schulman. *ACT UP Oral History Project*. Interview no. 173. 2 Feb. 2015. http://www.actuporalhistory.org/interviews/images/rollerena.pdf. Accessed 9 June 2018.

Román, David. *Acts of Intervention: Performance, Gay Culture, and AIDS*. Bloomington: Indiana UP, 1998.

———. "Remembering AIDS: A Reconsideration of the Film *Longtime Companion*." *GLQ: A Journal of Lesbian and Gay Studies* 12.2 (2006): 281–301.

Romero-Cesareo, Ivette. "Moving Metaphors: The Representation of AIDS in Caribbean Literature and Visual Arts." In *Displacements and Transformations in Caribbean Cultures*, ed. Lizabeth Paravisini-Gebert and Ivette Romero-Cesareo. Gainesville: UP of Florida, 2008. 100–126.

Rose, Malú Machuca. "Giuseppe Campuzano's Afterlife: Toward a Travesti Methodology for Critique, Care, and Radical Resistance." *Transgender Studies Quarterly* 6.2 (May 2019): 239–53.

Ross, Mirha-Soleil, dir. *Chroniques*. Vtape, 1992.

———. "Meal Trans." *YWCA* Folder F0033-3-5. Mirha-Soleil Ross Collection. Canadian Lesbian and Gay Archives. Toronto, Ontario, Canada.

———. "Preface." *Les Chroniques de Jeanne B. 1990–1993.* Folder F0033-2-25. Mirha-Soleil Ross Collection. Canadian Lesbian and Gay Archives. Toronto, Ontario, Canada.

———. "Reports (Meal Trans)." Folder: Reports (1 of 2) F0033-3-12 and Reports (2 of 2). F0033-3-13. Mirha-Soleil Ross Collection. Canadian Lesbian and Gay Archives. Toronto, Ontario, Canada.

Ross, Mirha-Soleil, and Xanthra Phillippa Mackay, dirs. *Gender Troublemakers.* Vtape, 1993.

Roth, Nancy L., and Linda K. Fuller. Introduction. *Women and AIDS: Negotiating Safer Practices, Care, and Representation,* by Roth and Fuller. Binghamton: Harrington Park, 1998. 1–4.

Ruiz, Maria V. "Border Narratives, HIV/AIDS, and Latina/o Health in the United States: A Cultural Analysis." *Feminist Media Studies* 2.1 (2002): 37–62.

Ryan, Benjamin. "Is It Time for the End of 'AIDS'?" *Poz Magazine.* 1 July 2015. www.poz .com/article/AIDS-terminology-27461-9306. Accessed 7 June 2018.

Ryosho, Natsuko. "Experience of Racism by Female Minority and Immigrant Nursing Assistants." *Affilia: Journal of Women and Social Work* 26.1 (2011): 59–71.

sachse, jes. "Crip the Light Fantastic: Art as Liminal Emancipatory Practice in the Twenty-First Century." In *Mobilizing Metaphor: Art, Culture, and Disability Activism in Canada,* ed. Christine Kelly and Michael Orsini. Vancouver: UBC Press, 2016. 198–205.

Sandahl, Carrie. "Performing Metaphors: AIDS, Disability, and Technology." *Contemporary Theatre Review* 11, nos. 3–4 (2001): 49–60.

Sawdon-Smith, Richard. "Art and Activism in the Age of AIDS." *AIDS/ART/WORK,* 30 May 2008, City University of New York. Panel presentation.

———. "Artists' Statement." *Art Pos(t)er/AIDS Pos(t)er.* www.aidscultures.com. Accessed 10 Nov. 2008.

Schulman, Sarah. *The Child: A Novel.* New York: Carroll & Graf, 2007.

———. *Conflict Is Not Abuse: Overstating Harm, Community Responsibility, and the Duty of Repair.* Vancouver: Arsenal Pulp, 2016.

———. "Dear PosterVirus, This Is Why You Mean So Much to Me." In *Art AIDS America,* ed. Jonathan D. Katz and Rock Hushka. Seattle: U of Washington P, 2015.

———. *The Gentrification of the Mind: Witness to a Lost Imagination.* Berkeley: U of California P, 2012.

———. "Interview with Carol Guess." *Lambda Book Report* 15.2 (Summer 2007): 16.

———. *My American History.* New York: Routledge, 1994.

———. *People in Trouble.* New York: Dutton, 1990.

———. *Rat Bohemia.* New York: Dutton, 1995.

———. *Stagestruck: Theater, AIDS, and the Marketing of Gay America.* Durham: Duke UP, 1998.

———. *The Ties that Bind: Familial Homophobia and Its Consequences.* New York: New Press, 2009.

Sears, Alan. "Queer Anti-Capitalism: What's Left of Lesbian and Gay Liberation?" *Science & Society* 69.1 (Jan. 2005): 92–112.

Sedgwick, Eve Kosofsky. *The Epistemology of the Closet.* Berkeley: U of California P, 1990.

Serano, Julia. *Excluded: Making Queer and Feminist Movements More Inclusive.* Berkeley: Seal, 2013.

Sevelius, Jae M., JoAnne Keatley, Nikki Calma, and Emily Arnold. "'I Am Not a Man': Trans-specific Barriers and Facilitators to PrEP Acceptability among Transgender Women." *Global Public Health* 11, nos. 7–8 (2016): 1060–75.

Shabazz, Rashad. "Mapping Black Bodies for Disease: Prisons, Migration, and the Politics of HIV/AIDS." In *Beyond Walls and Cages: Prisons, Borders, and Global Crisis*, ed. Jenna M. Loyd, Matt Mitchelson, and Andrew Burridge. Athens: U of Georgia P, 2012. 287–300.

Shakur, Assata. "To My People." 4 July 1973. Speech.

Sharpe, Christina. *In the Wake: On Blackness and Being*. Durham: Duke UP, 2016.

Showalter, Elaine. *Sexual Anarchy: Gender and Culture at the Fin de Siecle*. New York: Penguin, 1990.

——. "Syphilis, Sexuality, and the Fiction of the Fin de Siècle." In *Sex, Politics, and Science in the Nineteenth-Century Novel*, ed. Ruth Bernard Yeazell. Baltimore: Johns Hopkins UP, 1986. 88–115.

Simpson, Leanne. "Not Murdered, Not Missing: Rebelling against Colonial Gender Violence." Blog entry. *Nations Rising Blog: It Ends Here Series*. 5 Mar. 2014. www.leannesimpson.ca/writings/not-murdered-not-missing-rebelling-against-colonial-gender-violence. Accessed 8 June 2018.

Sinclair, Raven. "Identity Lost and Found: Lessons from the Sixties Scoop." *First People's Child and Family Review* 3.1 (2007): 65–82.

Singleton, Melinda. "Fighting for My Life." In *Women, AIDS, and Activism*, ed. the ACT UP/NY Women and AIDS Book Group. Boston: South End, 1990, 45–54.

Slade, Eric, and Mic Sweney, dirs. *Acting Up for Prisoners*. Frameline, 1992.

Smith, Ali. "Cold Comfort." Review of *Excerpts from a Family Medical Dictionary*, by Rebecca Brown. *guardian.co.uk*, 28 Feb. 2004. www.guardian.co.uk/books/2004/feb/28/biography.highereducation/print. Accessed 15 Nov. 2008.

Smith, Andrea. *Conquest: Sexual Violence and American Indian Genocide*. Durham: Duke UP, 2005.

Smith, Christopher. "Gettin' 'Down' with the 'Below': Visual AIDS 2016 and the Politics of 'Archival Activism': A Conversation with AJAMU." *AIDS and Memory*, special issue of *Drain*, with Amber Dean, ed. Ricky Varghese, 14.2 (2016). drainmag.com/gettin-down-with-the-below-visual-aids-2016-the-politics-of-archival-activism-a-conversation-with-ajamu/. Accessed 10 July 2017.

Smith, Susan Lynn. *Sick and Tired of Being Sick and Tired: Black Women's Health Activism in America, 1890–1950*. Philadelphia: U of Pennsylvania P, 1995.

Snorton, C. Riley. *Black on Both Sides: A Racial History of Trans Identity*. Minneapolis: U Minnesota Press, 2017.

Sontag, Susan. *Illness as Metaphor and AIDS and Its Metaphors*. New York: Picador, 1989.

Spade, Dean. *Normal Life: Administrative Violence, Critical Trans Politics, and the Limits of Law*. Brooklyn: South End, 2011.

Spiro, Ellen, dir. *DiAna's Hair Ego*. Women Make Movies, 1989.

Spurlin, William J. *Lost Intimacies: Rethinking Homosexuality under National Socialism*. New York: Peter Lang, 2009.

Stanford, Ann Folwell. *Bodies in a Broken World: Women Novelists of Color and the Politics of Medicine*. Chapel Hill: U of North Carolina P, 2003.

Stanton, Katherine. *Cosmopolitan Fictions: Ethics, Politics, and Global Change in the Works of Kazuo Ishiguro, Michael Ondaatje, Jamaica Kincaid, and J. M. Coetzee.* New York: Routledge, 2005.

Stepić, Nikola. "AIDS, Caregiving and Kinship: The Queer 'Family' in Bill Sherwood's *Parting Glances.*" *European Journal of American Studies* 11.3 (2017): 1–12.

Stevens, Lorraine, and Vera Hill. "Empowering the Poor." Box 17, folder 2 (AIDS in the Black Community). Joseph Beam Papers, *The Schomburg Center for Research in Black Culture.* Archives Division, New York Public Library.

Stockdill, Brett C. *Activism against AIDS: At the Intersections of Sexuality, Race, Gender, and Class.* Boulder: Lynne Reinner, 2003.

Stockton, Kathryn Bond. *The Queer Child: Or Growing Sideways in the Twentieth Century.* Durham: Duke UP, 2009.

Straube, Trenton. "COVID-19 Criminalization: Seven Lessons From the HIV Response." *Poz.* 30 Mar. 2020. https://www.poz.com/article/covid19-criminalization-seven-lessons -hiv-response. Accessed 22 Apr. 2020.

Strauss, Cee. "The Physical and Narrative Confinement of Ashley Smith: The White Female Victim in Prison and on the News." *The Indiscernible: The Department of Art History and Communication Studies,* 28 Apr. 2011, McGill University, Montréal. Conference presentation.

Stryker, Susan, dir. *Screaming Queens: The Riot at Compton's Cafeteria.* Frameline, 2005.

———. *Transgender History.* Berkeley: Seal, 2008.

Sudbury, Julia. "Introduction: Feminist Critiques, Transnational Landscapes, Abolitionist Visions." In *Global Lockdown: Race, Gender, and the Prison Industrial Complex,* ed. Sudbury. New York: Routledge, 2005. xi–xxviii.

"Surviving the AIDS Genocide." *People with AIDS Coalition Newsline* 38 (Nov. 1988). People with AIDS Coalition Records, 1987–1993. Manuscript and Archives Division, New York Public Library, Astor, Lenox, and Tilden Foundations.

Symington, Alison. "Criminalization Confusion and Concerns: The Decade Since the Cuerrier Decision." *HIV/AIDS Policy and Law Review* 14.1 (May 2009): 1–10.

Szott, Kelly. "Expanding the Mission of Harm Reduction: A Public Health Population and Its Members' Perspectives Towards Health." In *Critical Approaches to Harm Reduction: Conflict, Institutionalization, (De-)Politicization, and Direct Action,* ed. Christopher B. R. Smith and Zack Marshall. New York: Nova, 2016. 169–84.

Taylor, Darien. Interview by Alexis Shotwell and Gary Kinsman. *AIDS Activist History Project.* 7 Feb., 24 May 2014. https://aidsactivisthistory.files.wordpress.com/2016/06 /aahp_-_darien_taylor.pdf. Accessed 21 Nov. 2017.

Thom, Kai Cheng. *I Hope We Choose Love: A Trans Girl's Notes from the End of the World.* Vancouver: Arsenal Pulp, 2019.

Thorne, Jackie Evelyn. "Imperial Court Happenings." *Gulf Coast Transgender Community: An Outreach Organization* 8.1 (Jan. 1996): 6. Transgender Archives, University of Victoria. Victoria, British Columbia, Canada.

———. "Jet Trails." *Gulf Coast Transgender Community: An Outreach Organization* 8.5 (May 1995): 6. Transgender Archives, University of Victoria. Victoria, British Columbia, Canada.

Titchkosky, Tanya. *Reading and Writing Disability Differently.* Toronto: U of Toronto P, 2007.

Tomso, Gregory. "Bug Chasing, Barebacking, and the Risks of Care." *Literature and Medicine* 23.1 (Spring 2004): 88–111.

Tourmaline. "Last Year during Chloe Dzubilo's Memorial . . ." *The Spirit Was . . . .* 7 May 2012. *Tumblr.* thespiritwas.tumblr.com/post/22593369357/last-year-during-chloe-dzubilos-memorial-antony. Accessed 15 Sept. 2016.

"Toward an AIDS Archive." Blog entry. *Visual AIDS.* July 2017. https://www.visualaids.org/gallery/detail/1188. Accessed 28 Nov. 2017.

Transsexuals in Prison: A Newsletter for and by the Transsexual Offender. 1991. Transgender Archives, University of Victoria. Victoria, British Columbia, Canada.

Treichler, Paula A. *How to Have Theory in an Epidemic: Cultural Chronicles of AIDS.* Durham: Duke UP, 1999.

Treleavan, Scott. "Look After Each Other." *PosterVirus.* 27 Nov. 2013. *Tumblr.* postervirus.tumblr.com/search/look+after+each+other. Accessed 3 Mar. 2018.

Turner, Caitlin M., Jennifer Ahern, Glenn-Milo Santos, Sean Arayasirikul, and Erin C. Wison. "Parent/Caregiver Responses to Gender Identity Associated with HIV-Related Sexual Risk Behavior among Young Trans Women in San Francisco." *Journal of Adolescent Health,* 65.4, (2019): 491–97.

Turney, Robin. Interview by Alexis Shotwell and Gary Kinsman. *AIDS Activist History Project,* with Sri. 26 May 2014. https://aidsactivisthistory.files.wordpress.com/2016/06/aahp-robin-turney-sri.pdf. Accessed 17 May 2018.

Vaid, Urvashi. Foreword. *Hospital Time.* By Amy Hoffman. Durham: Duke UP, 1997.

Varghese, Ricky. "At 35: Writing the Viral Bildungsroman." *AIDS and Memory,* special issue of *Drain,* with Amber Dean, ed. Ricky Varghese, 14.2 (2016). drainmag.com/at-35-writing-the-viral-bildungsroman/. Accessed 10 July 2017.

Velasquez-Potts, Michelle C. "Regulatory Sites: Management, Confinement, and HIV/AIDS." In *Captive Genders: Trans Embodiment and the Prison Industrial Complex,* ed. Eric Stanley and Nat Smith. Oakland: AK Press, 2011. 119-132.

Vint, Sherryl. *Bodies of Tomorrow: Technology, Subjectivity, Science Fiction.* Toronto: U of Toronto P, 2007.

Vowel, Chelsea. *Indigenous Writes: A Guide to First Nations, Métis, and Inuit Issues in Canada.* Winnipeg: Highwater, 2016.

Wald, Priscilla. *Contagious: Cultures, Carriers, and the Outbreak Narratives.* Durham: Duke UP, 2008.

Walia, Harsha. (Panel speaker). "We Can't Police Our Way Out of the Pandemic." Zoom Meeting, 18 Apr. 2020. https://youtu.be/AK9ioHaTu38?t=1262. Accessed 25 Apr. 2020.

Ware, Syrus Marcus, Joan Ruzsa, and Giselle Dias. "It Can't Be Fixed because It's Not Broken: Racism and Disability in the Prison Industrial Complex." In *Disability Incarcerated: Imprisonment and Disability in the United States and Canada,* ed. Liat Ben-Moshe, Chris Chapman, and Allison C. Carey. New York: Palgrave Macmillan, 2014.163–84.

———. (Panel speaker). "We Can't Police Our Way Out of the Pandemic." Zoom Meeting, 28 Mar. 2020. https://youtu.be/j6s_FZu9F1s?t=4633. Accessed 25 Apr. 2020.

Washington, Harriet A. *Medical Apartheid: The Dark History of Medical Experimentation of Black Americans from Colonial Times to the Present.* New York: Harlem Moon, 2008.

Watney, Simon. "AIDS and the Politics of Queer Diaspora." In *Negotiating Lesbian and Gay Subjects,* ed. Monica Dorenkamp and Richard Henke. New York: Routledge, 1995. 53–70.

———. *Policing Desire: Pornography, AIDS, and the Media.* London: Continuum, 1997.

———. "The Spectacle of AIDS." In *AIDS: Cultural Analysis Cultural Activism,* ed. Douglas Crimp, Cambridge: MIT P, 1988. 71–86.

Watson, Julie. "*Autographic* Disclosures and Genealogies of Desire in Alison Bechdel's *Fun Home.*" *Biography* 31.1 (2008): 27–58.

Wein, Daryl, dir. Richard Berkowitz, perf. *Sex Positive.* Regent Films, 2008.

Wendell, Susan. *The Rejected Body: Feminist Philosophical Reflections on Disability.* New York: Routledge, 1996.

———. "Unhealthy Disabled: Treating Chronic Illnesses as Disabilities." *Hypatia* 16.4 (2001): 17–33.

Wesley, Sandra. (Panel speaker). "We Can't Police Our Way Out of the Pandemic." Zoom Meeting, 28 Mar. 2020. https://youtu.be/j6s_FZu9F1s?t=3392. Accessed 25 Apr. 2020.

Whitbread, Jessica. *It's Not a Secret: Women Build Communities.* Audio installation, McColl Center for Art and Innovation, Charlotte, North Carolina, 2014.

———. "Space Dates (With Morgan M. Page): Project Statement." *Jessica Lynn Whitbread.* jessicawhitbread.com/project/space-dates/. Accessed 10 June 2017.

Whitbread, Jessica, Jonny Mexico, and Theodore Kerr. "Love Positive Women!" *No More Potlucks* 43 (2016). nomorepotlucks.org/site/love-positive-women-jessica-whitbread -jonny-mexico-theodore-ted-kerr/. Accessed 17 May 2017.

"Why Has New York Failed . . ." *Village Voice* 2 Apr. 1985.

Wilson, Ciann L, Sarah Flicker, and Jean-Paul Restoule. "Beyond the Colonial Divide: African Diasporic and Indigenous Youth Alliance Building for HIV Prevention." *Decolonization: Indigeneity, Education & Society* 4.2 (2015): 76–102.

Withers, AJ. *Disability Politics and Theory.* Halifax: Fernwood, 2012.

———. *If I Can't Dance, Is It Still My Revolution.* 2014. stillmyrevolution.org. Accessed 12 Nov. 2014.

Wojnarowicz, David. *Close to the Knives: A Memoir of Disintegration.* New York: Vintage, 1991.

Wolfe, Maxine. "The AIDS Coalition to Unleash Power (ACT UP): A Direct Model of Community Research for AIDS Prevention." In *AIDS Prevention and Services: Community Based Research,* ed. Johannes P. Van Vugt. Westport: Bergin & Garvey, 1993. 217–48.

Women and AIDS Project. Newsletter. Winter, 1990. AIDS and Adolescents Network of New York records, Manuscripts and Archives Division, New York Public Library, Astor, Lenox, and Tilden Foundations.

Women and AIDS Resource Network (WARN) Records. AIDS and Adolescents Network of New York records, Manuscripts and Archives Division, New York Public Library, Astor, Lenox, and Tilden Foundations.

Wong, Laylani. "Community News: California AIDS Office Convenes First Transgender Forum." *Bay Area Reporter* 30 May 1996. GLBT Historical Society. San Francisco, California.

Woodland, Erica. "A Way Forward: Integrating Disability & Healing Justice into the HIV/ AIDS Movement." *Brown Boi Speaks,* 13 Nov. 2015. brownboispeaks.com/2015/11/13/a -way-forward-integrating-disability-healing-justice-into-the-hivaids-movement/. Accessed 15 Aug. 2017.

Woubshet, Dagmawi. *The Calendar of Loss: Race, Sexuality, and Morning in the Early ERA of AIDS.* Baltimore: Johns Hopkins UP, 2015.

Xhonneux, Lies. "Performing Butler? Rebecca Brown's Literary Supplements to Judith Butler's Theory of Gender Peformativity." *Critique* 54 (2013): 292–307.

———. *Rebecca Brown: Literary Subversions of Homonormalization*. Amherst: Cambria, 2014.

Yarborough, Melanie. "The Transgender and Gay Interface." In *Girl Talk*, ed. Powder Puffs of California, 12.6 (June 1997): 2. Transgender Archives, University of Victoria. Victoria, British Columbia, Canada.

Yee, Jessica. "Sustainable Justice through Knowledge Transfer: Sex Education and Youth." *Canadian Woman Studies* 28.1 (Fall 2009/Winter 2010): 22–26.

Youngblood, Stephanie. "Biomedical Nostalgia in Crisis." *AIDS and Memory*, special issue of *Drain*, with Amber Dean, ed. Ricky Varghese, 14.2 (2016). drainmag.com /biomedical-nostalgia-in-crisis/. Accessed 10 July 2017.

Index

academia, 12, 14, 18, 84

ACT UP, 10, 34, 155, 159; /LA, 101–102, 151–52; /New York, 32–32, 46–47, 49–52, 78; /San Francisco, 152; Oral History Project, 31–32, 46–47, 49–50, 100, 153–54; protests, 12, 83, 100–102, 152–53; social media, 45

Acting Up for Prisoners, 151–54

activism, HIV: as disability activism (*see* HIV: as disability); civil disobedience, 10, 12–13, 31, 49, 70, 107, 118 (*see also* ACT UP: protests; Stonewall Riots); defined as caregiving, 2–3, 5, 9–10; transnational, 133–34, 136–37

afrofuturism, 24. *See also* Butler, Octavia

AIDS Action Now! (AAN), 97

AIDS Activist History Project, 65; Oral History, 46–47, 97

AIDS Counseling and Education (ACE), 22, 151, 153–56

Ajamu, 37

Almeida, Shana, 17–18

American Medical Association (AMA), 98

anger, 49–50, 62, 79, 104, 135, 138

Annie Oakley's Girl, 117

anticapitalism, 2, 6–9, 16–20, 32–33, 71–72, 76, 88, 134, 141, 161

Anzaldúa, Gloria, 134

archives: absences in (*see* erased histories); ArQuives, 57; caring for, 6–7, 13–14, 36–38, 81–83, 161; GLBT Historical Society, 68, 160; Lesbian Herstory Archives, 8n, 54–55; New York Public Library HIV, 14–15, 32, 44, 53–54, 65, 68, 98, 154; as resistance, 65–67, 70; Smithsonian's Archives of American Art, 82; transmisogyny in (*see* transmisogyny: in HIV archiving); University of Victoria's Transgender Archives, 57

Army of Lovers: A Community History of Will Munro, 119–20

art, HIV, 12–13, 15–16, 35–39, 41–42, 65–67, 71–72, 81–83, 85–86, 120. *See also* video

asexuality, 109

Asian communities, HIV caregiving in, 69–70

assimilation: and confronting ableism, 2–3, 80; and homonormativity, 41, 44, 60, 109–10, 116, 141–43; HIV activism and kinship resisting, 54, 76; small press against, 70–72, 127

Auerbach, Nina, 25

autobiography, 2, 21, 44, 65–70, 76–77, 81, 97–104, 112, 117, 125–27; scholarship, 134–35. *See also* interviews; Kincaid, Jamaica; tumblr

Ayala, George, 78

Ball, Bradley, 32

ballroom, 38–39

Baynton, Douglas, 61

Beam, Joseph, 10

Bebushi: Blacks Educating Blacks about Sexual Health Issues, 10

Ben-Moshe, Liat, 130

Berkowitz, Richard, 39–40

Bernard, Kim, 46–47

About the Author

Marty Fink is an assistant professor in professional communication at Ryerson University.